'Til Death Or Dementia Do Us Part

MARILYN REYNOLDS

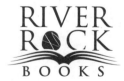

RIVER ROCK BOOKS

Published by:
River Rock Books
P.O. Box 19730
Sacramento, CA 95819

ISBN: 978-0-9994385-0-3

Cover art: Angela Tannehill, ThinkstockPhotos.com

Author photograph: Dick Schmidt

ACKNOWLEDGMENTS

I am ever grateful for the unwavering support of so many. These include Marg and Dale Dodson, Norman and Judy Franz, Kathy and Joe Harvey, Beth Reynolds, The Hundred Hours Club participants, Sharon Reynolds-Kyle and Doug Kyle, Matthew Reynolds and Leesa Phaneuf Reynolds, Jerry Reynolds, Marilyn and Bill Sandbom, and Jeannie and Bill Ward, and countless others.

My writing colleagues, including Karen Kasaba, Kathy Les, The Loft Writers, and the Noepe Workshop participants. Their close readings and shared insights were invaluable.

Those who, among others, worked to bring this book to fruition, including Jan Haag, Katie McCleary, Krista Minard, Julia Moore and Angela Tannehill.

The professionals who treated both me and Mike with respect, and who offered specific help when they could, and empathy when they couldn't. These include the staff at Accent Care Hospice Services, Dr. William Au, Dr. Patricia Brunner, Dr. Frank Capobianco, Carol Kinsel of Senior Care Solutions, Dr. Michael McCloud, and other nurses, physician assistants, and emergency hospital doctors, whose names are now lost to me.

The army of caregivers whose hard work and compassion helped ease the guilt and pain of "placement."

CAST OF CHARACTERS

Michael V. Reynolds, 1940–2014

Marilyn Reynolds (wife and narrator) 1935–

*****Sharon Reynolds Kyle** oldest child, 1958– (Previous Marriage)
   *Husband, Douglas Kyle, 1956–
   *Daughters, Subei Reynolds Kyle, 1995–; Lena Reynolds Kyle, 2001–

*****Cynthia Lynn Foncannon** (Cindi), second child, 1959– (Previous Marriage)
Daughter, Ashley DiFalco, 1991–
Son, Kerry Ryan Foncannon, 1993–
Kerry's Significant Other, Tara Collins

*****Matthew Michael Reynolds,** youngest child, 1969– (Birth Father, Michael)
Wife, Leesa Phaneuf-Reynolds, 1970–
Daughter, Mika Genevieve Reynolds, 2006–

*****Dale Eugene Dodson**, Marilyn's brother, 1944–
Wife, Margaret Jean (Pecoraro) Dodson, 1945–
Daughter, Corry Ruth Dodson, 1970–

Jerry Reynolds, Mike's brother, 1935–
Wife, Jackie Reynolds, 1938–
Daughter, Elizabeth Reynolds, 1961–
Daughter, Laura Sue Thompson, 1963–
Son, David Reynolds, 1968–

Hazel Virginia Piercy, Marilyn and Dale's aunt, 1919–2013
   Husband, Martin
   Daughter, Linda
   Wife, Barbara

* **Jeannie and Bill Ward**—Longtime friends, fellow travelers

*__Marilyn and Bill (1935–2013) Sandbom__—Marilyn Reynolds' friends since elementary school, Mike's friends by marriage. Longtime fellow travelers.

*__Kathy and Joe Harvey__—longtime friends, fellow teachers in Southern California.

*__Norman and Judy Franz__—longtime friends, Norman and Mike taught together in Southern California and remained friends for life.

The 100 Hours Club also included: Judy and Gerry Laird, Jo Souvignier and Rod Nystrom, Nancy and Bill Giachino, Barbara and Alan Lazar, Linda and Dave Dawson, and Don Ditmer, all stalwart friends whose generosity of spirit was remarkable.

*__Members of the "100 Hours Club,"__ which consisted of those who had taken at least 100 hours out of their daily lives to offer both practical and emotional support during these challenging times. They took Mike to lunch, to movies, on drives. They helped pack up the house, sold things on ebay and Craigslist, transported boxes of books to the Friends of the Library donation center, and a seeming ton of household items and clothing to Goodwill. They provided food on workdays. They followed and responded to my FTD blog. They lifted my spirits and Mike's, too, back when his spirits could be lifted.

Mike's Southern California music friends who also offered positive support over the past years: **Bill Schmidt, Nancy Obrien, Jeannie Davenport, Mary Rawcliffe, Lou Robbins, and others.**

With the exception of **Carol Kinsel** and her organization, **Senior Care Solutions**, all names of doctors, caregivers, and residential facilities have been changed.

FOREWORD

After 13 years of being a primary care doctor, I have had the distinct honor of caring for many wonderful people with dementia of all kinds. Dementia is an awful, frustrating disease that leaves patients, caregivers and physicians feeling powerless and sometimes hopeless. At a certain point in the progression of dementia, when patients are no longer capable of knowing where they are or who is around them, there comes a shift. I have found the care that is most needed then is for the patient's loved ones who struggle with the changes and sense of loss as dementia smothers the person who the patient once was.

"'Til Death or Dementia" is a love story above all else, a wonderful account of the relationship that Marilyn Reynolds celebrated with her husband, Mike. It is beautiful to read and an example of what I hope for all my patients' families—a deep reflection on memories representing all that was wonderful before the diagnosis of dementia. These memories can bring joy amid the struggle with the realities of the disease. In a most courageous way, Marilyn shares her feelings, doubts, fears and regrets as she recalls Mike's personality and cognitive changes, both before and after his dementia diagnosis. Her words convey the emotional roller coaster in a way that the reader can feel every turn, loop, climb and freefall. Her remarkable ability to share serves as a road map for all those who care for someone with dementia, as I have witnessed among hundreds of families.

I would hope that everyone would read this story, not just those who find themselves caring for someone with dementia. This beautiful book reminds us that life is finite and worth living to the fullest. It brought a renewed mindfulness for me that every moment counts, and despite all life's challenges, love reigns supreme and can carry us through the darkest of times. Our legacy lives on in those we leave behind. Read this book, then think about the life soundtrack you want, and start singing!

Christopher Lillis, MD FACP
Medical Director for Primary Care Transformation
UC Davis Health, Sacramento, California

PROLOGUE

In July 2009, after 42 years of marriage, my 69-year-old husband, Michael Reynolds, was diagnosed with frontotemporal dementia (FTD). As frightening and horrendous as that diagnosis was, it went a long way toward explaining the frustrating and puzzling changes in Mike's behavior that I'd been experiencing from as early as 2005.

Neither I nor any of our family members or friends had ever heard of frontotemporal dementia until the term was applied to Mike. Upon delivering the diagnosis, the neurologist explained that FTD is a neurodegenerative disease. It affects the frontal and temporal regions of the brain—regions that control personality and social behavior, reasoning, speech and language comprehension, and executive functions. There is no known cause. No cure. It is progressive, but the rate of progression is unpredictable. Aricept and/or Namenda, drugs often used to slow the onslaught of Alzheimer's disease, might in some cases slow the progression of FTD, though that, too, was uncertain.

We were certainly aware of Alzheimer's. The Alzheimer's Association estimates that 60 to 80 percent of all cases of dementia result from Alzheimer's disease. Vascular dementia, caused by inadequate blood flow to the brain, which often occurs with strokes, accounts for 20 to 30 percent, FTD perhaps 10 to 15 percent. In comparison to the wealth of Alzheimer's publications and media reports widely available, information about FTD was scarce and required a degree of diligence to uncover. I, our grown children, my brother and sister-in-law, and some in our close circle of friends, set about gathering and sharing whatever information we could find. While we familiarized ourselves with whatever FTD information was available, we watched Mike increasingly embody classic textbook symptoms.

This account of the steady deterioration of a much loved, bright, talented, funny, emotionally connected husband, father, brother, uncle, music colleague, and friend is unavoidably skewed by my own particular view. But, particular as it is, it also depicts much that is common to victims of FTD and to the ones who love them.

For those whose lives are being turned upside down by FTD, I hope this account of our experiences opens a window onto the emotional and practical tasks ahead. If such tasks are behind the reader, I hope there may be some comfort in knowing that he or she is not alone with the pain, sadness, frustration, guilt, resentment, and loss that inevitably accompany this journey.

Marilyn Reynolds
Sacramento, California

WHO MIKE WAS BEFORE HE WASN'T

From *The Sacramento Bee*, December 28, 2014

Michael Vance Reynolds passed away peacefully this past December 19. Born to Lindsay Crawford Reynolds and Leeta Reynolds in Artesia, New Mexico, in 1940, he grew up in Tampa, Florida. In 1965, after receiving a graduate degree in Church Music from Southwestern Seminary in Fort Worth, Texas, he moved to the Los Angeles area, where he began his career as a teacher and singer, and where he met and married Marilyn Dodson Klick.

For 26 years Mike taught choral music in the Alhambra School District, first at Mark Keppel High School, then San Gabriel High School. He was beloved by both students and faculty. Mike sang professionally with the Los Angeles Master Chorale, the Roger Wagner Chorale, and other Los Angeles area groups, joining them on tours throughout the United States, Canada, Russia (then the Soviet Union), Israel, Japan, Estonia, Latvia, Lithuania, and England. He was tenor soloist at the First Presbyterian Church of Hollywood (1976–81; 1989–95) and All Saints Episcopal Church in Pasadena. After retiring from teaching, he and Marilyn relocated to Sacramento where he took a position as music director at the Unitarian Universalist Society of Sacramento, directed the Chanteuses vocal ensemble, sang with Camerata California, and with other Sacramento groups. One of his favorite musical endeavors was performing, with two other close musician friends, the music of Yip Harburg/Harold Arlen, Noel Coward, Cole Porter, and Stephen Sondheim. He was known not only for his sensitive and poignant interpretation of familiar songs, but also for his rousing, comic renditions of "Lydia the Tattooed Lady," and "Mad Dogs and Englishmen."

Mike loved family and home, movies and books, and enjoyed many warm and close friendships. He and Marilyn, along with other family and friends, traveled together to Great Britain, Italy, France, Mexico, and through much of the United States. Some of their favorite travel experiences were on various walking tours in England, Ireland, and France. For the last several years, Mike lived under the cloud of frontotemporal dementia. The family wishes to thank the many caregivers, counselors, and friends who provided comfort and assistance.

In addition to Marilyn, his wife of 47 years, Mike is survived by his three children, Sharon Reynolds-Kyle, Cindi Foncannon and Matthew Reynolds; five grandchildren, Subei and Lena Kyle, Ashley and Kerry Foncannon, and Mika Reynolds; and also by two brothers and several nieces and nephews.

A service celebrating Mike's life will be held at 2 p.m. on Saturday, Jan. 10, 2015, in the sanctuary of the Sierra Arden United Church of Christ, 890 Morse Ave., Sacramento. A reception will follow in Pilgrim Hall. Gifts to honor Mike's life may be given to The Association for Frontotemporal Degeneration, Radnor Station Building 2, Suite 320, 290 King of Prussia Road, Radnor, PA 19087, or to the Unitarian Universalist Society Building Fund: 2425 Sierra Blvd., Sacramento, CA 95825.

REMINDERS OF THE RICHNESS
OF LIFE BEFORE FTD

January 10, 2015

The service was, appropriately, filled with music. Subei and Lena sang that old Beatles song, "In My Life." Francisco, a college sophomore and Subei's boyfriend since high school, provided a flawless, sensitive piano accompaniment. Everything was layered. I was watching our beautiful granddaughters, hearing them sing tenderly and in harmony, and I was also seeing Mike, hearing him sing the same song many years ago at Norman and Cindy Franz's wedding—Norman, Mike's loyal friend who had come up from Southern California with his present wife, Judy, to be a part of our sad/happy festivities.

The last verse of "In My Life," repeated twice, was a struggle for Subei and Lena to sing through smoothly. No one was unmoved. I was gripped by all that had been and all that was lost. The lyrics speak poignantly of never losing affection for people and things from the past and ends with the memorable line: "In my life, I love you more."

Linda Dawson, who had accompanied Mike at many past performances, worked her piano magic.

Bill Schmidt played "Morning Has Broken" on the organ. I'd requested that, not only because Mike and I had both liked the old Cat Stevens version, but also because I was beginning to get a sense, as the song says, that "Mine is the sunlight, mine is the morning ..." after such a long darkness. I couldn't help thinking that Mike, too, had been lifted from the dark imprisonment of his broken brain.

I was the first of the family to speak. I welcomed all who had come to celebrate Mike's life, and thanked family and friends who had walked that arduous journey with us, then went on to say, among other things:

Mike and I were extremely fortunate to have had 38 enriching and fulfilling years together. We were married for 47 years, but the first 38 are the ones I'm remembering today.

Mike's gifts to me were many and varied. The warmth of his ongoing love, his dedication and devotion as husband and father, his interest in our home environment— building decks, brightening patios, bringing in flowers, painting and wallpapering. Well … maybe wallpapering wasn't such a welcome gift, but all the rest were.

And there was the great gift of his humor. Many years ago, halfway across the Atlantic on a flight to London, guidebooks piled on our pulled-down trays as we considered what we were about to see and do, Mike took my hand, looked deep into my eyes, and said, "My main goal on this trip is to make you laugh until you wet your pants." That in itself nearly did it.

Our personality differences could hardly have been more extreme. I was logical and practical to a fault. Mike lived by intuition and spontaneity. As you might guess, that was sometimes challenging. But we held a core of common values that went beyond personality styles. We valued family, friendship, education, intellectual and emotional growth. We valued a connection to the broader world. We shared music, books, movies, hopes, dreams, disappointments and frustrations, every aspect of our lives. We brought each other to worlds neither of us would have experienced on our own, and in the process, we each were stretched and deepened.

Even with the responsibilities of family and the demands of teaching high school music, Mike never put his commitment to singing and performing professionally on the back burner. He made room for whatever opportunities came his way—LA Master Chorale, opera chorus, soloist in church choirs and synagogues, and working on original shows that featured works from what we've come to think of as "The Great American Songbook."

Honestly, although I respected Mike's decisions when he took unpaid leaves from teaching in order to tour far away places with one or another choral group, I wasn't always wild about the effects such decisions had on the home front. I wasn't always wild about night after night of rehearsals for one or another performance, either, but I delighted in the outcomes. It was pure joy seeing and hearing Mike in action, whether with a formal choral production, either singing or conducting, or hamming it up with Bill Schmidt on a song and dance routine, proclaiming that only "Mad Dogs and Englishmen" go out in the noonday sun. It was a pleasure to listen as he practiced one or another song, to talk with him about possible interpretations. To cheer him on.

When my long-dormant desire to write more than shopping lists bubbled up through the hard-packed shell of practicality, I didn't give it much credibility. Wife, mother, teacher, daughter, movies, books, living in the world—how would I ever eke out enough time to develop a writing life?

But ... there was Mike, a daily living example of one who nurtured his own creativity, and "eking out" was not what he did. In this area of my life, sometimes to his chagrin, he became my role model.

Although Mike respected my decision to take an unpaid leave from teaching in order to finish a book, he wasn't wild about the temporary cut in income. The same was true when I went off for three weeks to a writing retreat in Vermont. But, as I loved the results of his music practices, he loved the results of my writing practices. His insights and critiques of first draft materials were invaluable. He was backup at conference book sale tables. He cheered me on.

Without Mike's sometimes challenging example, I could easily have put writing on the back burner and let daily practicality rule. Instead of having 12 published books in print, I could easily now be wondering, what if I'd finished that first book attempt, instead of going to the market, or picking up the cleaning. It was the inspiration of Mike's dedication to music that gave me the resolve to write and keep writing, especially when the pesky details of the practical world worked so hard to draw me away.... I am grateful for all that we brought to each other....

Next, Sharon told of how, at the age of 8, soon after she started taking piano lessons from "Mr. Reynolds," she began seeing him more often when he dropped by our house. She began noticing that her mom was having long conversations on the phone with him. She told of the gifts of talent and broader experiences he brought to our little band of three. She read "In Blackwater Woods," by Mary Oliver, that speaks of the beauty of nature, the ubiquity of loss, the necessity of love, and the essential task to let go when the time comes.

For the previous five years, all of us who loved Mike had been working on the task of letting go. Maybe we finally could.Cindi didn't speak during the formal part of the service, but just days after Mike's death she posted a touching online tribute to him, complete with pictures and music. Many, many of Mike's former students also posted online tributes.

Matt finished the immediate family segment of the service, offering a "behind the scenes" account of Mike's life as he knew it:

Since my dad died a few weeks ago, I've been combing through the family archives, looking at photos and scanning images for the slideshow that will be playing in the reception hall. As you can imagine, this has been a bittersweet process. Nevertheless, I have noticed a couple of themes, the most obvious of which has been his life onstage, performing, directing, singing.

Of course, even in those pictures where he's not onstage, he was still often performing. He had a way of always being "on." The camera inevitably compels performance. No surprise—we tend to photograph those moments we hope will be worth saving, worth looking back on. But it's a little uncanny how my dad seemed to have an awful lot of these moments worth remembering. This was a VERY well-documented life.

My favorite—a picture of him from 1954, in Tampa, with the Royal Palms Orchestra, age of 14 dressed in his white dinner jacket, standing at the mic in front of a big band orchestra.

But I also want to acknowledge that there was another side to my dad. He was a complex human being.... One of the many things I loved about him was his silliness. He loved corny jokes and never failed to make himself and others laugh during a round of charades.

He could also be judgmental. I won't talk so much about that today....

He was an incredible teacher who inspired so many of his students and challenged them to take on ridiculously ambitious pieces of choral music. I had the privilege of teaching some of his students when I occasionally substituted at San Gabriel High School and heard firsthand about the impact he had on so many lives. And yet he ALWAYS COMPLAINED about his job. He never failed to express his misery about having to start a new week or having to go back after summer break.

He was deeply religious but constantly questioned the rigid dogmas he was exposed to in the various churches he was affiliated with. And while his spiritual growth was an enormous part of his life, he was without doubt one of the most materialistic people I've ever known. This was a man WHO LOVED HIS STUFF! He obsessed over his Royal Doulton figurines, his china and silver, his clothes, his shoes, his Waterford crystal. His favorite places of worship were not only All Saints, Hollywood Presbyterian, and the Wilshire Temple, but Bullock's, Jacob Maarse, and Nordstrom.

One of the hardest things to watch over the last four years was the cruel transformation of this complexity into one-dimensionality.... I will never be able to forget the agony I felt every time I made the long drive to, first, Carmichael Oaks, then Porto Sicuro, then Sister Sarah's, then Green Hill. I'm terribly sad I wasn't able to be by his side when he *left this earth, but I'm relieved I didn't have to see him at the last institutional facility.*

I also need to say how utterly grateful I am to the two people who worked the hardest behind the scenes to make sure Dad was well cared for and as comfortable as it was possible for him to be. Marg, and especially Mom, thank you. Dad was incapable of expressing or, to my knowledge, experiencing gratitude towards the end, but I know he would want me to thank you for him. I'm not sure if heaven exists, but if it does, there is a special place there for the two of you.

Even though these last few years have been so hard, there are still moments and fragments that I will cherish. The last time I saw him, this past August, most of my time with him was spent watching him shuffle past me on the perpetual loop he walked in whichever facility he was in. Every couple of passes, I could catch his eye and smile and say, "Hi, Dad." I could hold out my arms and he would walk over to me and open his arms to me, and we would give each other a big hug, and I could tell him I loved him.

Looking at photos, I see a life VERY well lived. I see a PUBLIC person who loved and was very well loved. But I'm also grateful for the life behind the scenes, for those fragments of connection during even the most difficult times—for all the practice and hard work that made the performances seem so effortless.

Growing up, one of my favorite memories is waking up to the sound of his voice on Sunday morning. But it wasn't a song or piece performed in its entirety. It was the exercises he would sing to warm up his voice. I could hear him down the hall of our house in Altadena, sitting at the piano in the living room, singing his own unique version of scales. This was my Sunday morning soundtrack.

So here, in honor of my dad, in memory of my experience of him behind the scenes, in the spirit of his willingness to look silly, and MOST ESPECIALLY, with apologies to you for having to listen to this, I'd like to sing a snippet of the Sunday morning song.

To the surprise of all who knew him, Matt then sang the first five notes of a scale up and back. I would guess it to be C,D,E,F,G,F,E,D,C.

After Matt spoke, our niece, Corry, sang of lingering "Precious Memories,"
How they ever flood my soul
In the stillness of the midnight
Precious sacred scenes unfold.

I wished Mike could have stayed around long enough to see Corry's development as a singer/songwriter.

Dale, Marg, Jeannie, Norman, Mary Rawcliffe, and Bill Schmidt, all had stories to tell. Stories of kindnesses. Stories of Mike's shared gifts of music. Laugh-out-loud stories. So many bittersweet reminders of what we were all missing.

Bill accompanied Mary on the piano as she sang a Noel Coward song that starts, "I'll see you again, whenever spring breaks through again…", conjuring memories of the shows they and Mike had done together at the Pewter Plough in Cambria, or Valhalla at Lake Tahoe. If I ever feel the need to collapse in sobs, I'll listen to our recording of that piece.

Bill played a medley of songs from Mike's 50th birthday show, "Ages, Stages and a Few Laughs." Roger, the present UUSS minister, read comments of appreciation from students that had come in the mail or been posted on Facebook. There was a tribute from Barbara Lazar, expressing the joys of making music with him. The Chanteuses singers did a rousing rendition of "Down by the Riverside," a piece Mike had led them in many times. They followed that with "Sing Me to Heaven." It was beautiful and heartfelt, and although several singers were tearful, their sound was spectacular.

For the final hymn I chose "For All the Saints," which, although it depicts a theology neither of us subscribed to beyond adolescence, is strong and rousing, and conjures other times and other memorials—and particularly conjures Mike's voice from Marg's father's memorial all those many years ago.

We invited everyone who had ever sung with Mike, or sung under his direction, to come to the front and lead the congregational singing. They lined the series of broad steps leading to the level of the pulpit and crowded several rows deep in front of the first pews. Bill gave a short introduction on the organ, and the assembled group sang out. Their voices filled the sanctuary. There was no other word for it but "glorious."

A few closing words from Roger, then Bill put the organ through its paces, belting out a jubilant Irish jig, a postlude in keeping with Mike's joy of dance, and music, and celebration.

Somewhere in the depths of joys and sorrows flooding through that time of assembled remembrances, Mike came back to me. He had been gone for such a long time, in such a strange way, and my interactions and attentions to the remnant of him overshadowed the Mike who had once been.

"Welcome back," I whispered to the lingering Mike.

"COME BACK TO SORRENTO," OR "TOMA A SURRIENTO"

2005

It is August 2005. We are in Sorrento, Italy, at L'Antica Trattatoria, a small restaurant, off the beaten path. In the soft glow of candlelight, our half-empty wine glasses rest on a crisp white linen tablecloth. A serenading violinist plays in the background, "Come Back to Sorrento." We laugh that the scene is, except for us, like something out of a movie. Me, nearly 70, and Mike 65, we don't exactly fit a movie image of romantic leads. Still, on this, our 38th wedding anniversary, we are romantic.

"Here's to us," Mike toasts with the Campania recommended by our waiter. "I'm so glad we found each other. I can't imagine life without you."

As we tap glasses, I quote the inscription I'd so long ago had engraved inside the ring that was to be Mike's. "With love deepening, enduring,"

Over a long, slow dinner, we talk of shared good times and bad.

I mention our honeymoon. Two days alone in the mountains, then a trip to Florida to meet Mike's family. My two daughters, Sharon, 9, and Cindi, 7, went with us.

"Remember how my mother insisted we take their bedroom—the one without a door?" Mike says.

We laugh, remembering that the only room in that whole house with a door on it had been the bathroom, making the bathroom our honeymoon suite.

"I think I may still have a bruise on my back from the bathtub faucet," I say.

After the tagliolini for me—with lemon cream sauce, red prawns, and lumpfish on creamed spinach, and equally lofty lamb chops for Mike, after sipping Limoncelo and hearing yet one more plaintive rendition of "Come Back to Sorrento," we walk the few blocks back to our hotel. It's a balmy night, lit by a bright half moon, seasoned by a sweet bay breeze.

Getting ready for bed, Mike sidles up to me, kisses me lightly on the back of my neck and asks, "Wanna do it in the bathtub? Just for old time's sake?"

"Let's forgo the challenge of intrusive plumbing fixtures and make use of our comfy rented bed," I say. And we do.

A few days later we take the train to Rome, where we meet up with the Dodsons—my brother, Dale, sister-in-law, Marg, and their grown daughter, Corry. The next day we meet my cousin's wife, Janice, and her 11-year-old granddaughter, Taylor. I no longer remember the details and surprises of our Rome meeting. I wish I could. What I'm left with is the sense of miscommunications, chance meetings, and light-hearted laughter. Well … I do remember the Colosseum and the Vatican. The Spanish Steps and Santa Maria Trastevere, a church dating from the third century. Mostly though, I remember fond, shared laughter, coupled with a sense of wonder that we were actually in Italy, that we had all found each other in Rome.

After a few days in Rome, and with a few wrong turns, Mike and I in one rented car, the Dodsons in another, Janice and Taylor on a combination of trains and buses, we all manage to find our way to Montepulciano, where our daughter, Sharon, son-in-law Doug, and their two children, Lena, 5, and Subei, 11, are already ensconced in the picturesque villa Sharon had ferreted out online. When we arrive in the late afternoon, they are outside, sitting at a big round wooden table, shaded by two large trees the owner later identifies as "Umbrella Pines." Quick hugs all around. Quick chatter of travel adventures. Luggage taken to individual accommodations. Quick uses of the facilities, and then we are all at the big table, in the yard that overlooks a rolling hill of grapevines. Doug opens wine, Sharon puts cheeses and bread rounds on the table, and we catch up with one another's travel adventures.

We fall into a loose, unspoken practice of side trips from Montepulciano every morning. In small, ever-changing groups, we stroll through out-of-the-way villages. We visit Florence, so overwhelmed by the art that we make peace with the knowledge that we won't see it all, that it's better to experience a few pieces deeply than to impart on a self-imposed survey course. Mike and I join the group that, sensibly, hires a driver for the narrow, curvy, cliffhanging drive overlooking the Amalfi Coast. But wherever our day trips take us, we gather in the late afternoon, around the big wooden table, with whatever day's accumulation of wines and cheeses we've found along the way. Laughing at mishaps, showing our wares, and always the ongoing back and forth with what has become this precious sabbatical from worries for our troubled world, the weighing and measuring of where and when to go for dinner.

On the last night in Montepulciano, with only Dale and Marg and Mike and me left at the villa, in honor of our just-passed anniversary, Dale and Marg take us to dinner at a local restaurant. Mike and I married almost exactly one year after Dale and Marg tied the proverbial knot. We married in the same church, with many of the same guests, and always, either in person or from a distance, we mark each other's anniversaries.

I don't remember the name of the restaurant, or what it looked like inside, though I think there were candles. I don't remember what we ate, though I think we agreed it was one of the best meals ever. Beyond any of those details, though, here's what I do remember: We are sitting at an outside table, on a high balcony, with a panoramic view of the night sky that is unhampered by tall buildings or rooftops. The bright, full moon is huge, breathtaking, shining on our little table, shining on us, as if we alone have been singled out for its radiance. Now, years later, as I sit writing of that night, I sense again the gravitational pull of that brilliant, Italian moon.

Back home in Sacramento, timed to coincide with the next full moon, Mike and I treat the Dodsons to a different sort of anniversary dinner. Jeannie and Bill Ward join us for the celebration on the Fair Oaks footbridge that spans the lower banks of the American River. We set up a card table and six of those folding canvas chairs, like the ones you see lining the fields of youth soccer games. Eschewing paper and plastic products, Mike covers the well-worn card table with a white tablecloth and a small bouquet of yellow roses. By the time the others join us on the bridge, the table is set with "real" plates and wine glasses. A pre-cooled bottle of Chardonnay nestles in one of those cylindrical marble wine chillers, and a red is opened and breathing.

Our food offerings—salads, both green and potato, fried chicken, chocolate chip cookies for desert—are not of a Montepulciano style. Nevertheless, it is a tasty meal, worthy of the Dodsons' 39th anniversary festivity. In between stories and remembrances of the history of their years together, others who've come out on the bridge to enjoy the full moon, or who are simply walking from one side of the river to the other, pause to remark on our dinner set-up and to ask about the occasion. Mostly younger, the friendly passersby express awe and wonder when they learn that the featured couple are marking 39 years. That is, in turn, a source of amusement to us.

With the darkening sky and the rising full moon, we sing moon songs. Mike and Marg are clear and loud enough that Dale, the Wards, and I, can sing out without danger of hurting any passing listener's ears: "Blue Moon," "Shine on Harvest Moon," "It's Only a Paper Moon," "Moon Over Miami," and, finally, "Moon Up In the Sky," a song written and composed by Mike's Aunt Treval, who for decades dreamt of success in the music business while working as a telephone operator in Marble Hill, Missouri.

August 2005 was packed with good times. Then came September and hints of trouble ahead. As hints came more frequently, as hints became certainties, no matter how many times I listened to "Come Back to Sorrento," with Mario Lanza's resonant tenor voice, backed by a full orchestra replete with weeping strings, I knew beyond a doubt we could never return to Sorrento.

January 2010

Dear Mike,

I know this letter, and all of the letters I've written to you since 2009, are only pretend, that you will never read them, that even if someone were to try to read them to you, you couldn't listen. But it is strangely comforting to be telling parts of this story directly to *you, rather than simply telling it* about *you.*

The worst part of this most difficult time of my life is that I'm not able to talk through any of it with you. Not the loss of our home, not the endless work of taking care of you, not the bankruptcy process, not having to live with almost no discretionary income. All of that is difficult, and not what I expected to be dealing with in my 70s. But not being able to talk with you, to share my deepest thoughts and feelings with you—that is the very worst. For most of our 40-plus years of marriage we were each other's closest confidantes. Late at night, over dinner, in front of the fireplace, in bed in the mornings, we talked, laughed, worried, reassured. There were times we argued angrily over who knows what. But nearly always, our home was a loving home, our bed was a loving bed, and we laughed. I miss that all so much. I miss your arms around me. I miss the warmth of love in your eyes. I miss your frequent, spontaneous compliments—"You're a pretty woman, Marilyn," or "Your lips look delicious!" I don't think such compliments will come my way again.

I am ever grateful to be surrounded by friends and family who care for us both, who travel alongside me on this sad, uncharted odyssey, who offer help at every turn. Still, I hunger for your loving support and insights, for the depth of conversation that was once ours together.

Loving you to the end,
Marilyn

'TIL DEATH OR DEMENTIA DO US PART

I COULD WRITE A BOOK

Fall 2005

It is September 2005. Sometime between that glorious August vacation in Italy, and my 70th birthday celebration the following month, something shifts. Mike, usually Mister Party Organizer, is strangely uninvolved in preparations for my September 13 birthday party—my 70th—leaving the planning of the food, drinks, program and decorations to others.

Dale and Sharon gather pictures and stories. Doug scans the photos, adds music, and puts together a slide show that spans all 70 years of my life. It is funny and poignant, and when finished, Doug tells me, "I now know more about your life than I do my own." But where is Mike in all of this?

He's said he'll take care of the wine for the 40 or so people who will be joining us in the big banquet room at the Newport Beach Dunes Resort. I've chosen the venue for its proximity to an area that was a significant part of my growing-up years.

As the party date grows closer, and Mike's still not done anything about the wine, Sharon offers to purchase it for him. He likes that idea. She knows what wines will work best and where to get good deals. She can buy the wine, and Mike will pay her back. Before the party, Sharon gives Mike the receipts for the wine. He tells her he'll write a check. He doesn't. I remind him that he needs to reimburse her. He says he will, but it doesn't happen. It's unlike him. Weeks later, after several reminders, I write the check from my own account.

Mike's contribution to the party program was to sing "If They Asked Me I Could Write a Book," a song that over the past several years had gained meaning for us. Mike saw the whole book idea as a connection to my late-blooming writing career. The last lines about making two lovers of friends were reflective of our very early history together. Many songs had meaning for us, but this came as close to being "our" song as anything else.

He sang beautifully and with great feeling, holding my gaze with those last lines, "And the simple secret of the plot, is just to tell them that I love you, a lot.

Then the world discovers as my book ends, how to make two lovers of friends." It was sweet and reassuring, but I continued to be puzzled by his relative indifference to details of the whole celebration. With most husbands this might have been business as usual, but it was definitely not business as usual for Mike. Looking back, I think that was when frontotemporal dementia made its first foray into the essence of Mike, starting the long and torturous assault on his capacity to listen, to empathize, to think logically, to participate in meaningful conversation, to love. At the time, though, it simply seemed that his love for me was waning. In those first FTD days there were still times when he was his most loving and connected self. But then, inexplicably, he would become distant and unreachable. After 38 strong years, was our marriage falling apart?

Revisiting that time, I realize that our 2005 financial practices should not only have raised a red flag, but should have moved me to fight long and hard to change our spending habits. We were overusing credit cards—the trip, my birthday bash, dinners out, Mike's habit of buying a new silk tie to wear to church every Sunday, season tickets for the San Francisco Symphony, which included overnights at our favorite boutique hotels, etc., etc., etc. It worried me that we were not quite coming out even at the end of every month. I'd always had a clearer vision of the big picture of our finances than Mike did, and I knew it was time for significant cutbacks. Cutting back, though, was not in Mike's nature, and I too easily let things slide.

The Italy trip had been an indulgence. It alone was not responsible for our ultimate financial downfall, but it was the beginning of a pattern. And although I may regret the pattern, I am ever grateful to remember Mike as he was in Italy: funny, witty and kind, sensitive and loving.

In the late '80s, when Mike was the tenor soloist at a large Episcopal Church in Pasadena, I attended regularly. I respected the church's social justice work, I loved the music, and I loved the poetry of the readings and prayers. I loved that all hymns and readings had been carefully adapted to contain inclusive language, but that the rhythm of the adaptations remained true. As long as I approached the service on a metaphorical rather than a literal level, it was meaningful to me.

Every Sunday, before communion, the priest announced that, "Wherever you are on your journey of faith, you are welcome at this table. All are welcome at Christ's table," and so, although I was not a believer, I regularly participated in the ritual of communion. For me, the process was not a statement of belief but rather recognition that I had a place in an ongoing human community, that we were all, the whole of humankind, in this mess of a world together.

As I held my hands out to receive the wafer, the priest often said, "The body of Christ, the bread of heaven," but sometimes it was "strength for the journey." The memories of my time with Mike in Italy became a source of strength for the long, rough journey ahead.

PANIC ATTACK OR...?

Winter 2005

U nlike a lot of writers, I don't keep a regular journal. I wish I did. I have somewhere between 15 and 20 potential journals of varying sizes and configurations, ranging from cheap composition exercise books with lined paper to hand-sewn, leather-bound journals with acid free paper made from sustainable forest pulp. No matter. They all have several entries for January of whatever year it was that I had resolved to keep a journal. Some of them have occasional entries as late as mid-February. Since I'm more likely to keep a trip record, some of the stashed journals have details of certain travels. Not one of them, though, offers a consistent record of any year of my life.

Now, having confessed my slovenly journal habits, it should come as no surprise that I can't be certain of the time frame of this event. I'm pretty sure it was sometime between the spring and winter of 2005.

Mike had followed closely the development of the Walt Disney Concert Hall, delighted to see that Los Angeles would finally have a world-class performance venue. In 1987, Lillian Disney, widow of Walt Disney, donated $50 million for the project. Although Frank Gehry completed the designs in 1991, between added costs and difficulty raising additional necessary funds, the building was not completed until 2003. According to my backup fact checker, Wikipedia, the Disney Hall grand opening was one of the most successful grand openings of a concert hall in American history. Shortly after the opening, Mike sat in on a rehearsal and fell in love with the place. He was itching to sing in the new concert hall.

From 1972 until we moved north in 1998, Mike had sung with the Los Angeles Master Chorale. He was no longer a regular with them, but he did occasionally go to LA to sing in a concert as a ringer when the tenor section needed bolstering. When, in 2005, the director of the Chorale called to say they needed help in the tenor section for an upcoming concert, Mike couldn't have been happier. He sent his tux to the cleaners. He cleaned and buffed his black patent leather shoes. Since he would only be there for one rehearsal, he looked over the music and practiced the most complicated sections.

The day before the rehearsal Mike flew to LA to spend time with singer friends he'd missed after leaving town. He called home right after the rehearsal, telling me the sound was glorious and raving about the beauty of the building. He was thrilled to be a part of it all. He called again the next night, a bit earlier than expected.

"How was the concert?" I asked.

"I couldn't do it."

Although Mike had never been fond of standing on risers for an hour or more, crowded by singers to his right and left, front and back, he'd done it in thousands of concerts in the U.S., Eastern Europe, Western Europe, Japan, Israel, and, I'm sure, others that would be listed in my journals, if I'd kept journals.

"Sweat was pouring off me. I felt faint. I had to get out of there!"

He'd made his way off the risers and to the side exit during the last number before intermission. At intermission he told the director he had to leave. He went back to his hotel room, called me, then spent a sleepless night before catching his early morning flight back home.

A long time friend and fellow Master Chorale singer encouraged Mike to try a beta blocker for next time. It worked for her. She reminded him that in his 30-plus years of singing with the chorale in a myriad of venues, the Disney Hall experience was the only time he hadn't performed perfectly. He should call the director. It didn't need to be the end of his Master Chorale experiences. But, embarrassed, afraid the same thing would happen again, he was through.

Whenever he spoke of that experience, which wasn't often, he always talked about the crowded, narrow risers, and said he got claustrophobic.

I knew how unusual and disturbing that experience had been to Mike. But it never occurred to me that it was anything other than a one-off panic attack. Now, though, I wonder if it was part of the onset of FTD.

THESE SHOULD BE
GOOD YEARS

2006

Mike had battled depression off and on for decades. He sometimes tried to get relief with an antidepressant, or help from a therapist, or both. And although life was not easy for either of us at his lowest points, there were plenty of moments of lightness, and there was consistently more light than dark. Then, in late 2005, early 2006, indifference and darkness were becoming more the norm. And, frankly, I was pissed.

We were no longer tied to full-time teaching jobs. We each had meaningful work, Mike as music director at UUSS and also with various other music projects and professional singing jobs. I was working on *No More Sad Goodbyes*, the ninth book in my Hamilton High series of teen fiction, and doing occasional author visits to schools, teacher workshops, and conference presentations. Still, our schedules were flexible enough for overnights in San Francisco, or with Sharon and her family in Woodacre. We visited Matt and Leesa in LA and were happily anticipating the birth of their daughter. Our home in Gold River was spacious and inviting—an easy place for friends and family to gather. We were financially secure.

These should have been very good years for us, but I was finding it more and more difficult to deal with Mike's dissatisfaction. He didn't like Sacramento. He wasn't appreciated at the church. He was upset with the direction Cindi's life was taking. He hated George W. Bush. Bush's arrogance with his misguided determination to drag us into a war with Iraq, the horrible loss of American lives and even more Iraqi lives, seemed to both of us to be criminal. I didn't disagree with Mike's assessment of our president and his cronies, but his over-the-top ranting was wearing. One time, after hearing Mike's litany of all that was wrong with his life, I accused him of robbing us of the great pleasure of our retirement years that was easily within our reach. "Sorry!" he'd said in a way that meant "leave me alone" rather than that he was truly sorry.

All I knew then was that the love and support I had so long felt from Mike was waning. The potential goodness of this stage of life was being sucked away by his negativity. If only I had known that Mike's brain was doing him wrong, I could have been more patient, more empathic. At least that's what I like to think. But I didn't know, and the more self-absorbed and distant Mike became, the more resentful I became. Because being resentful was not something I commonly experienced, I even resented becoming resentful.

Although the balance between good times and bad times was tipping, a scattering of moments of love and lightness were still within reach. I still held hope that a change in meds would ease things, or that some change of circumstances would help, or that a therapist would ask the questions that would lead Mike to a happier state.

Although Mike often displayed either disinterest or dissatisfaction with me, he was still a totally dedicated grampa—gentle, playful, funny. He loved little children, and he especially loved our grandchildren. I also loved them wholeheartedly, but my grandparenting style, like my personality, was less effusive and more practical than Mike's. We were a good balance. A good team.

When Sharon and Doug brought 4-month-old Subei home from China in 1995, we were determined to be as big a part of her life as we already were in the lives of Cindi's two children—Ashley (5) and Kerry (3). They'd always lived within easy driving distance, and we frequently visited back and forth. Maintaining regular contact with Subei would be more of a challenge, since she lived 400 miles away. Still, we planned to see this new baby at least every six weeks. The 800-mile round trip from Altadena to Woodacre was demanding, but getting to know that amazing little Subei creature and having her get to know us would be well worth the effort. One of the main reasons we moved north in 1998 was to be close enough to Subei to be a regular part of her life, too. And although Sacramento was still 100 miles from where Subei, Sharon, and Doug lived in Woodacre, a 200-mile round trip was a whole lot easier than the 800-mile round trips we'd been making from Altadena.

For the previous 30 years, ever since Dale and Marg had moved to Sacramento, we'd been visiting the capital city at least once or twice a year. Our longtime friends, Jeannie and Bill Ward, lived in Fair Oaks, part of the greater Sacramento area. On one of our trips north, we followed an open house sign into Promontory Point, a "village" in Gold River. We liked the house. The price was right. It was not more than 2 miles from the Wards', 20 minutes from Sacramento and the Dodsons', and an hour and a half from Subei, Sharon, and Doug.

The house we'd been living in in Altadena had been built in 1935. That was the same year I'd been built and, like me, it was needing more and more maintenance. The Gold River house was much newer and had obviously been well-maintained. Modern appliances! A roof guaranteed for the next 30 years!

On the drive back to Southern California, Mike and I hashed and rehashed the pros and cons of such a move. How would it be to leave longtime friends? How would it be for Mike to leave music friends? How would it be for me to leave my longtime writing group? Well, it wasn't as if we were moving to another country. When I asked Mike how he'd feel about leaving the Chorale, he said he was more than ready. He was tired of blending.

Before we signed on the dotted line for the house in Gold River, we talked with Cindi about the possibility that she and her kids might also make a move. We could help if she was willing. She was more than ready for a change and so jumped at the chance. Within two months of our move to Gold River, she, Ashley and Kerry had moved into a duplex just a few miles from our place. Still in close proximity to the first two grandkids, not close, but at least closer, to Subei.

In 2002, we'd gone to China with Sharon, Doug, and Subei, where they completed adoption arrangements for Lena, then 10 months old—another thrilling addition to the grandkid population.

On April 18, 2006, Mika Genevieve Reynolds, Matt and Leesa's daughter, was born at Cedars-Sinai Medical Center in Los Angeles. Sometime around the 14th, when it appeared that Leesa was in the beginning stages of labor, we made the trip south. It turned out to be one of those start and stop labors that are so frustrating, especially to the mother. Maybe the baby, too. Mika has not yet revealed her version of the event.

By the morning of the 17th, it seemed that birth was imminent. Then it wasn't. Then it was. Then it wasn't. Finally, when monitors showed the baby was experiencing some distress, a quick decision was made for a cesarean.

As I write this, a series of images come to mind—Leesa and Matt walking the halls of Cedars-Sinai, hoping to move labor along. Leesa, uncomfortable and unwieldy, laughing as we approached, remarking about early signs of stubbornness in this baby. Matt walking beside her, growing more concerned with each slow-passing hour.

I see me with Mike, at lunch, an outdoor, street-side table, within view of the hospital, both cell phones at the ready. And then, shortly after lunch, there was a healthy baby Mika, an exhausted Leesa, and a greatly relieved Matt. We were thrilled with this new granddaughter. Mike didn't think he could possibly love Mika any more than he loved the other grandchildren, but he allowed as how the "bone of my bone, flesh of my flesh" was an added bonus to his connection with Mika.

In 2006, even though things between us were fraying at the edges, Mike was still at his best with the grandkids.

In the realm of occasional times of love and lightness, season symphony tickets took us to San Francisco on a fairly regular basis. On symphony evenings we usually stayed overnight at Inn at the Opera, a small hotel, quaint and friendly, and an easy walk to Davies Symphony Hall and to favorite restaurants. The morning after the symphony we would make our way to Golden Gate Park. Often we would make use of our membership to visit the de Young Museum. At other times we wandered the gardens, stopping for tea in the Japanese Tea Garden. These were still invariably happy times for us. I worked to remind myself of the good times whenever Mike became distant and inconsiderate. Such work had become more demanding by the end of 2006.

Besides becoming less connected and more disgruntled, Mike had stopped doing any kind of exercise and had developed what might have been labeled a beer belly, except that he didn't drink beer. I tried to convince him to get back on a workout routine, reminding him that he always felt better when he was exercising and physically active. He gave lip service to the idea, but regular exercise for him seemed to be a thing of the past. Had he become unable to maintain a schedule? To follow an exercise plan? Possibly. He was not yet having any obvious problems keeping appointments or maintaining a choir rehearsal schedule. But a new plan? Was that already beyond him?

I wish I'd not been so caught up in my own unmet needs that I was missing subtle signs of a disintegrating brain. I wish I had been able to talk with Mike without arousing his defenses. I wish I'd not so often responded to Mike out of a sense of being wronged.

December 2012

Dear Mike,

Yesterday I went with a friend to see "Quartet." I thought so much of you, how you delighted in participating in the quartet that for so many years gathered to sing the high holidays, and in the occasional quartet formed by the soloists at Hollywood Presbyterian for a special program. I thought of you in the Master Chorale, in the concert version of "West Side Story," and the funny schtick you did with "Mad Dogs & Englishmen" and on and on. I think you would have loved the music, and Maggie Smith, and so much more.

The soundtrack was beautiful. A major theme running through the movie had to do with a performance of "Rigoletto" that the principals had done in their younger years, so there was a lot of la donna è mobile. Also included was Libiamo Ne Lieti from La Traviata and many more that I couldn't have named but that you could have.

Of course, it stirred up all kinds of dormant memories and emotions for me, hearing such wonderful music that I no longer hear without you to put on the CD or arrange for a trip to the symphony. I vowed to go through the still-packed box of your classical CDs and bring them in to sit beside Willie Nelson, and Johnny Cash, and Dolly Parton, and others from the first box of music I unloaded.

The scenes that brought me to tears, though, were the comic scenes from "The Mikado" of "Tit Willow" and "The Flowers That Bloom in the Spring." I remembered your San Gabriel High School production of "The Mikado." Talk about blood, sweat, and tears. But you made it happen. What a great success for the stage crew, the orchestra, and, of course, for you and your singers! Those bits took me back to that long lost time. I do so wish you had been able to live out your life in a manner similar to that depicted in "Quartet."

I go along day by day in my necessarily reinvented life, with you hovering at the edge of my consciousness. Then something, this time "The Mikado," brings your vivid memory to life, where I must let you linger for a moment. And then I lose you all over again.

Goddamned FTD. I miss you terribly.
Marilyn

IS THE MUSIC DIRECTOR'S JOB THE PROBLEM?

2007

There were several puzzling incidents during the course of 2007. Looking back over it now, a more obvious pattern of increasing cognitive difficulties emerges, but at the time I attributed such incidents to our growing frustration with one another, and to Mike's dissatisfaction with his work at the Unitarian Universalist Society of Sacramento.

Mike's undergraduate and graduate degree was in Church Music, and for most of his life, in addition to teaching and singing professionally, he'd held one church job or another, either as Music Director or as tenor soloist. He was Music Director from 1965 to 1972 at Temple City Christian Church, which is where we first met and where we were married in 1967.

As a professional musician, Mike wasn't particularly concerned with the theology of a church. He'd sung with a very conservative Presbyterian church in Hollywood, a very liberal Episcopal church in Pasadena, and for 10 or more years he sang high holiday services at a Los Angeles synagogue.

When we moved from Southern California to the Sacramento area in 1998, we went church shopping. Our hope was to find a place with a strong music program and with a theology that fit our belief systems. Although Mike had been raised and educated as a Southern Baptist, he'd long ago discarded the rigid literal interpretation of the Bible. I had not been a believer since my teen years.

For a short while in Southern California, when Mike was between church jobs, we'd attended a Unitarian Universalist church in Pasadena. We both appreciated the theology there. The music was good. The building was beautiful. It was a good fit for both of us. But when Mike signed on as tenor soloist with the large Presbyterian church in Hollywood, our days of being in the same space on Sunday mornings were over.

Now, starting fresh in a new area, it made sense to seek out the one denomination that had resonated with both of us. The Unitarian Universalist Society of Sacramento (UUSS) fit that criteria and within a year or so of moving we became members.

We respected people and organizations that were Christ centered. As the adapted cliché goes, some of our best friends were Christians. But we were definitely more at home with the UU's affirmation of "a free and responsible search for truth and meaning" than we were with the prescribed belief system that was a part of our earlier religious experiences.

At UUSS we'd found a fit. We formed friendships, hosted gatherings, participated in small group activities and, for the first time in 30-plus years, we were involved together in a church community.

The theology worked. The music less so. Although we basked in the freedom of unencumbered Sundays, Mike's frustration with what he perceived as sloppy music led him to sign on as UUSS Music Director when that job opened.

Musicians loved working with Mike. Within months of his start as Music Director, the choir had tripled in size. The congregation heaped praise on the enlivened music offerings. One of the UUSS choir members told me recently that Mike was the best director he'd ever sung with.

There were a number of accomplished musicians who were UUSS members, but they had not been involved with the music of the church. Mike found them, or they found him, and soon they were participating as soloists, or in special programs. Musicians from the broader community also took part in some of the more demanding works presented as part of the annual music festival.

Although the music program was thriving, by 2007 Mike was complaining often and loudly to me about all that was wrong at the church. The building was more of a multipurpose room than a sanctuary. There was no defined space for the choir. When there were only 10 singers that wasn't a problem. But finding a place for 30 singers was more complicated. The natural place was front and center, but that crowded the minister. The choir was sometimes in front, off to one side or the other, but that was not acoustically satisfying. Mike's opinion was that it was a more effective arrangement for the choir to sing from the center and for the minister to move to the side. The minister didn't agree.

They tried being on the stage. That had its own problems as singers became less attentive during the course of the sermon, as their posture became less than upright or, worse still, they nodded off. The choir was not happy with that arrangement, and Mike hated having them on display on stage. "This is a worship service, not a show!" he'd complain.

As was his habit, Mike maintained good spirits with his fellow musicians, but his private complaints to me were gaining force.

Mike hated meetings, hated being required to attend them. That was nothing new. He'd hated meetings as long as I'd known him. As a teacher he'd hated faculty meetings, department meetings, and budget meetings. As a choral conductor or professional singer in any number of churches throughout the years, he saw meetings as a waste of his time. What was new was not his attitude toward meetings, but the intensity of his indignation over being expected to attend.

Although I was the major recipient of his rants, there were one or two other UUSS workers with whom Mike shared some of his frustration. I realized that I was not the only one who was tiring of complaints when I stopped by the music office and saw that the custodian had taped a sign over Mike's desk:

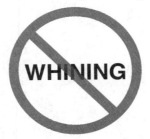

I considered such a sign for our family room but doubted it would be met with the same good humor as the music office sign had been.

After upwards of a year of wrestling with the possibility of leaving his post, Mike sent a letter to the board, stating his intent to resign effective January 31, 2007. In spite of being concerned about the loss of $18,000 to our yearly income, I encouraged Mike's resignation. Perhaps, without the frustrations of the church job, the cloud would lift.

In his resignation letter Mike expressed his appreciation for the choir and for other musicians of the congregation. He said, "It has been my great pleasure to work with the Music Committee," and named the two chairs he'd worked with during his time at UUSS. This was the same committee whose meetings he ranted on and on about having to attend. I expect there was truth in both of these responses, parts he loved, parts he hated. But I was only getting the hate side of things, and I had grown weary of the tirades.

IS IT HOT IN HERE?

2006–2007

In the spring of 2006, a grandmother in Texas had skimmed through the book her granddaughter was reading and was so shocked by what she read that she marched into the girl's middle school library and demanded that the book be permanently removed from circulation. The offending book was *Detour for Emmy*, a teen pregnancy story that is part of my "True-to-Life Series From Hamilton High." She also demanded that all of my other books be taken out of circulation. Of course, the grandmother had every right to monitor her granddaughter's reading, at least if the granddaughter's parents agreed. But it was outrageous to think she could ban certain books from the whole student body.

The middle school librarian had a comprehensive challenge policy in place and also had the support of the school's principal. As per policy, the book was read by members of the community, a minister, parents, business people and other educators. They ultimately decided, unanimously, that the book was appropriate for middle school readers and it stayed on the shelves. But this was not before an enormous brouhaha that had made the Dallas/Fort Worth 7 o'clock news for a full week.

In addition to the Texas challenge, there had been several other *Detour for Emmy* challenges during 2006. There are always a few. Over the years there've been challenges in Tennessee, South Carolina, Arizona, Illinois, and California, and probably many more that I don't know about. On the cover of each of my teen fiction books is the statement "True-to-Life Series from Hamilton High." So, teen pregnancy? Realistic? Yes, Emmy and her boyfriend had sex.

The other books in the series are also sometimes challenged. Nearly always they meet the challenge and stay on the shelves, and the news media are not involved. But between the Texas grandmother and other challenges, *Detour for Emmy* ended up in the No. 6 slot on the 2006 American Library Association's Top Ten Most Frequently Challenged Books list.

Mike couldn't have been more amused and proud of my growing reputation among certain circles as a writer of dirty books, a writer who was leading the youth of our nation astray. He happily spread the word to friends and colleagues that I had joined the ranks of others whose books had been banned—Mark Twain, Toni Morrison, Maya Angelou, Dr. Seuss, Maurice Sendak, Judy Blume, and on and on. What good company I was keeping! Hosted by the American Library Association, Mike accompanied me to Chicago where I, along with many others, spoke at the 2007 annual ALA Banned Books Week event. Mike was charming, totally engaged.

In addition to attending ALA events, we spent an afternoon at The Field Museum of Natural History. We marveled at the huge Cloud Gate sculpture in Millennium Park. We enjoyed dinner at some famous but now forgotten restaurant. But within a day of returning home, Mike was again dissatisfied and unhappy. It was beginning to seem as if it took a getaway for Mike to find any pleasure in life.

At home, what I was hearing from Mike was depression and discouragement. Try as I might, I couldn't get past my own take on life to have total empathy for him. I couldn't help feeling that his constant repetition of all that was wrong in his life, and his near total neglect of whatever was right, was partly to blame for his state of mind. Plus, I was tired of hearing it. One day, after a litany of complaints, I asked, "Is there anything, ever, you can enjoy or feel good about?"

"Of course," he said.

I asked that we spend just 15 minutes each day telling each other about whatever good had occurred during the previous 24 hours. We could do it when we had our pre-dinner glass of wine, I suggested. He agreed.

The first evening of our new ritual I expressed several things for which I was grateful. When it was Mike's turn he managed to comment that Sunny looked nice when he picked her up from the groomers, that he'd liked that I'd gone to breakfast with him that morning, and he was looking forward to the symphony. Our combined "goods of the day" lasted about five minutes before Mike shifted into complaining about a neighbor.

"Our 15 minutes isn't up yet," I told him, laughing. "No complaining for another 10 minutes!" I pointed out the window to the flowering plum tree. "Look how beautiful that is."

We somehow managed another 10 minutes. I thanked Mike, telling him how much I needed to hear some of the good stuff. We kept to the ritual a total of three nights. On the fourth night he said, "I don't want to do this anymore."

"I do," I said.

"It feels phony to me. I'm not playing that game," he said, and that was the end of it.

How could I stay with a man who was either incapable or unwilling to offer me even 15 minutes a day of positive conversation? On the other hand, maybe he needed an adjustment in meds? Maybe we should take a trip? Maybe if he could get a long-talked-about solo show going?

Looking back, it seems I was already the frog in the warming pot of water, not registering the gradually increasing heat, in danger of waiting until it was too late to jump, already bound for the soup factory.

YIP HARBURG?

2007

Mike had often performed songs with lyrics by Yip Harburg and, in doing so, became intrigued by the man and his works. This prolific lyricist was mostly unknown to the general public. Mike would tell audiences that whether or not they knew his name, most of them were certainly familiar with dozens of Yip Harburg's songs. Besides having written the lyrics to all of the "Wizard of Oz" songs, he was also the lyricist for "Paper Moon," "April in Paris," "Happiness Is Just a Thing Called Joe," "How Are Things in Glocca Morra," "Brother, Can You Spare a Dime," and hundreds more.

Once free of his UUSS music director responsibilities, Mike started work on a show that would focus solely on the music and life of Yip Harburg. He delved more and more deeply into Harburg's music and history with a zeal befitting a potential biographer. He told friends, fellow musicians, family, neighbors, and the clerk at our local dry cleaners how Yip Harburg had grown up on New York's Lower East Side, a community made up mostly of Russian Jewish immigrants. Yip had sat next to Ira Gershwin in school, and they discovered a shared interest in Gilbert and Sullivan. Gershwin took him home to his "swank" apartment and played "H.M.S. Pinafore" for him on the Victrola. This was around 1911 when Yip was only 15 years old. He later wrote that from that time forward he was tied to Ira Gershwin.

Mike also often told of Harburg's social activism, much of which came through in his lyrics. His "Brother, Can You Spare a Dime" had become a touchstone for the downtrodden during the Depression. Besides his music, Harburg was also active in progressive political organizations—active enough to be blacklisted during the McCarthy era.

As much as I, too, loved the work of Yip Harburg, I sometimes felt that Mike was monopolizing too much of the conversation when we were with friends. But he was a good storyteller and brought plenty of energy to whatever he was saying. I hoped it was only my imagination that eyes sometimes became glazed with yet one more story, or one more repetition of a Yip Harburg story. I was aware that it was not only me with whom he was listening less and talking more.

At first Mike's plan was for a one man show in which he would portray Harburg. Then he thought it might be good to bring in a soprano to add vocal interest. Soon he was collaborating with a director, pianist, eight or more singers and a few local actors.

Although I was working to meet a deadline for my book *No More Sad Goodbyes*, I offered to help Mike and the director come up with a script for the show. Over our many years together, Mike and I had collaborated easily in a number of ways. I always sought Mike's take on any writing project in process. He was an astute and insightful reader, able to point out what more was needed and what was redundant, to note the strengths in a manuscript and see what needed clarification. He might say, "I'm not sure Lynn would give in so easily here," or simply, "I don't know what's going on here." My books were better than they might have been because of Mike's close readings.

Conversely, Mike had consistently sought my take on choices of music and how things fit together in a program. Did it make more sense for the third song to be last? Did there need to be a more lively number between the two ballads? Did his introduction say what he wanted it to say?

So we started on a script. Mike and I listed aspects of Harburg's life that we wanted to be sure to include and songs Mike particularly wanted to feature. I wrote a rough draft of how that might work. The director met with us and quickly envisioned ways in which the show might be staged. Mike talked with other singers about joining in. Mike and the director decided to include a quartet of singers that would function as a kind of Greek chorus. We revised the script. The project kept growing and, to me, it seemed to grow more unwieldy with each passing day. We revised again. When we finally got what seemed to be close to a last draft, I hightailed it back to my office to finish *No More Sad Goodbyes*. But I took hope from the positive interactions Mike and I had during our script writing process.

There were changes in the cast—who would sing which part, who would stand where. Rehearsal times were always in flux, trying to accommodate musicians with other commitments. Rehearsals with the whole group were in evenings, but a few of the key players, Mike, the pianist, and the director, were often able to work in the afternoons at our home. Music, talk of programming, possible clothing, lighting, staging, all seeped through the doors of my office as I struggled to finish my manuscript on time. I began taking my laptop to the library, Starbucks, a park. These were not particularly quiet places, but the noise was not my noise and, although I loved "How Are Things in Glocca Morra," I found it to be much more distracting than whatever might be playing at Starbucks.

Although Mike was enthusiastic and upbeat during Harburg rehearsals and related meetings, he was either distant and uninvolved with me, or using me as a sounding board to express whatever anger he was feeling—maybe anger at a neighbor, or the treatment of gays and lesbians. His continued rants against George Bush and Cheney and Rumsfeld were frequent and vitriolic. I didn't disagree with the content of Mike's tirades, but the heat of his rage began to seem less about the Bush administration and more about Mike's need to rant. One evening, in a crowded restaurant, Mike's loud and heated Bush-critique ended with, "If I had a gun, I'd shoot George Bush!"

A few people looked over at our table then, fortunately, went back to their meals.

Back home that evening I tried to impress on Mike the dangers of threatening the president with bodily harm. His only response as he turned and walked away from me was, "Well, *someone* should shoot him."

I don't know which was worse, the anger, or the depression. I remember one morning in particular. It was around 10 o'clock or so, and I had just started working on what I hoped would be final revisions for *No More Sad Goodbyes*. Mike came into my office and flopped down in the big, leather chair opposite my desk. He let out a long sigh.

"I'm soooo discouraged," he said.

"What about?"

"I'm just discouraged!"

"Can I help?"

"No! I'm going back to bed!"

With that he stomped upstairs. Later, when I went up to our bedroom to ask if he wanted to come down for lunch, he said he wasn't hungry. He just wanted to stay in bed. The only place in the world he felt safe was in his bed.

Over dinner that evening, Mike's mood slightly better, I asked if I might call for an appointment for him to see Dr. Carlson, our primary care physician.

"Why?"

I mentioned a few recent times when he'd said he wasn't feeling well, and other times when he'd been terribly depressed. It couldn't hurt to get things checked out.

Because I knew the happy face he always put on for doctors, when the day of the appointment arrived, I asked if I might go with him.

"Sure."

As was his pattern, when Dr. Carlson asked how things were going with Mike, he was all smiles. Everything was going great.

"What brings you in today?" she asked.

"Marilyn wanted me to see you."

Dr. Carlson asked me about my concerns. I told her that several times recently, Mike had complained of not feeling well, that he sometimes went back to bed after breakfast, that he was often depressed.

Dr. Carlson ordered blood work, prescribed an antidepressant, Cymbalta, and gave Mike a referral to Dr. Bertoli, a cognitive psychologist. Maybe help was on the horizon.

Mike took the Cymbalta religiously. He saw Dr. Bertoli regularly. He remained cheerful and upbeat with friends and continued to be mostly angry, depressed, and distant with me.

May 22, 2013

Dear Mike,

Today is your birthday. 73. I visited you yesterday, though "visit" doesn't exactly describe the activity. You were in the house when I got there, in the hallway on your way out the front door, to continue the trajectory of your seemingly compulsive loop. I say seemingly compulsive because you did pause for a moment to give me a smile and a hug, a millisecond kiss on the lips. You spotted the cookies I'd brought in a baggy. Do you expect that routine now? Look for them? I don't know, but you were eager to get one, and I handed it to you. A great big yummy-looking chocolate chip cookie from Trader Joe's bakery. It made my mouth water just to look at it, but I am on my seemingly eternal quest to lose 10 pounds—it's always 10 pounds, a reachable goal—and I restrained myself from gobbling the second cookie in the baggy. You reached for that one on your next round and I handed it over. You took a bite, then set it on the hallway table, picked up the first cookie you'd taken a bite from and continued your loop.

On your next round I handed you the birthday card I'd picked up at the dollar store. I used to be so careful with your cards, picking up first one, then another, maybe making a special trip to that midtown store that has enough choices to keep one busy for hours. I looked for the perfect picture, the perfect message, then took great care in the note I added on the inside. I know you used to do that, too. Today I grabbed something colorful that said "Happy Birthday," added a quick "Love, Marilyn," sealed the envelope and wrote your name on the front.

On your third round I gave you an enthusiastic "happy birthday" and handed you the card. You opened half the envelope, set it on the hallway table, took another bite of your cookie and continued your incessant trajectory. Next round you picked up the card, opened the envelope the rest of the way, left it on the table, picked up the remains of one of the cookies, set it on a shelf on the way back through, etc., etc., etc. Tedious, isn't it? Tedious to write about. Tedious to read about. How much more tedious must it be for you?

I don't spend much time wishing, and my wishes aren't big. But I do wish you could sit still long enough for me to sit next to you on the couch and tell you I've done the best I can, and that I'll be watching out for your care and comfort for the duration.

I know these letters are fruitless, but maybe as looping is your compulsion, writing to the now nonexistent you is mine.

Remembering better birthdays,
Marilyn

DESPERATE FOR
A GOOD TIME
2007

Mike and I had taken our first Wayfarers walk back in 1990. We'd gathered a group of friends for a weeklong walk in the Cotswolds. Traveling in England before the walk, then being guided through beautiful countryside and quaint villages, walking along with friends and having the luxury of relaxed time for extended conversations, was a remarkable experience. We were hooked on The Wayfarers. A few years later many of the Cotswolds' group got together for a Wayfarers walk in England's Lake District. In 1996, after exploring/enjoying Paris, we walked through the Burgundy wine area of France. In 1998 we did another Wayfarers walk in the Ring of Kerry area of Ireland. Mike's music colleagues, also good friends, Bill Schmidt and Nancy Obrien, joined us on that trip.

Now, in 2007, in an effort to lift Mike's spirits and to try to pull us together, I'd signed us up for another English Wayfarers walk, in Dorset along the Jurassic Coast. I knew the trip was a financial stretch when I'd sent in the deposit. Then, with the loss of Mike's UUSS income, the expenses of the trip became more of a plunge than a stretch. But I was desperate for positive experiences with Mike and barreled ahead with plans for the trip.

In August, we met Bill Schmidt in London and from there drove to Rye where we'd booked three nights at The Mermaid Inn. Paris, the Lake District, Ireland, Germany—wherever we'd been there were places we'd dreamed of returning to "some day." I suspect that's a common traveler's dream. The Mermaid Inn was one of those rare dreams come true. The inn was established in the 12th century and rebuilt in 1420. The hotel and the town of Rye were full of history, and Mike, something of an Anglophile, was in his element.

The three of us had a delightful stay in Rye. Besides being rich with romantic, historical lore, Rye is also a place of natural beauty, just 2 miles inland from the English Channel, at the confluence of three rivers. We climbed the steep and narrow steps of St. Mary's bell tower, then an old ladder leading to the roof, where we had a stunning view of Rye rooftops, the surrounding countryside, the rivers, the sea. From that vantage point it seemed that all must be well with the world.

Four days later, the welcoming Wayfarers dinner at the Fairwater Head Hotel in Hawkchurch defied the stereotype of tasteless English food. Freshly caught and nicely prepared local fish, fresh vegetables from the garden, and some kind of toffee pudding that I wolfed down, telling myself the next day's 8-mile walk would take care of the extra thousands of calories. As had been the case with every other Wayfarers walk, the leader (Muff) and the manager (Yannick) were both charming and knowledgeable.

The morning started with a full English breakfast and an easy walk to a manor where the gardens had been restored to the original 1920s design. The gardener led us past the grass tennis court, fountains, the large kitchen garden and "reflection" areas. He told us the "lady" was pleased with the house because, unlike their previous manor, this one had "only" nine bedrooms and was quite manageable—with servants, of course. After lunch Mike returned to the hotel saying he wasn't feeling well. Bill and I continued on with the group to visit a former monastery with 900 years of history to its credit.

The next morning we visited Lyme Regis where the scene of Meryl Streep, wrapped in a big cloak, standing at the end of the Cobb was filmed for "The French Lieutenant's Woman." The weather was dark and the atmosphere as moody as it had been in the film. We were quite taken with it. Again, after lunch, Mike went back to the hotel, and Bill and I walked on. When I got back to the room in the late afternoon, Mike was napping. I showered, then woke him for dinner. He complained of not feeling well and dragged around until we got downstairs, where he immediately brightened and turned on the charm. After dinner Mike, with Bill at the hotel piano, sang several of Yip Harburg's songs. They ended with "When the Idle Poor Become the Idle Rich," which asks how we'll determine who's poor and who's rich when everyone has ermine, and plastic teeth. "And when all your neighbors/are upper class/You won't know your Joneses from your Ass-tors."

The clever lyrics, Mike's delivery, and Bill's piano acrobatics left the gathered audience laughing and clamoring for more.

I, too, enjoyed their performance. They were, as always, relaxed and interactive with the audience. Both consummate performers. But I was finding it more and more difficult to reconcile the Mike I experienced in private with the charming public Mike.

Not once on the Wayfarers part of our trip did Mike complete a full day's walk. He might sleep in in the morning, then join us for lunch and the afternoon trip. Or go back after lunch with Yannick while the rest of us walked on. I brought him aspirin, felt his head, brought him tea. Asked what more I could do for him. What was wrong? He just didn't feel well.

I don't remember now what set it off. We were in our room at the hotel, getting ready for dinner. We, with the exception of Mike, had walked shady, wooded paths to beautiful gardens with panoramic views of the sea. I was telling Mike some of the high points. "I'm sorry you're missing so much of this," I said.

"I don't feel well!"

"I know. I'm sorry."

Mike pulled a clean shirt from his suitcase and turned to face me. I could tell by his scowl he was angry. I wasn't sure why.

"I want to spend the rest of my life with someone who likes me!" he shouted, seemingly out of the blue.

"I want that, too," I told him.

"Much of the time I have the feeling that you don't even like me!" he said.

"I often feel that with you, too," I said. Then I added, "I do like you. I love you. I totally love the wonderful, caring, funny, good listener, good friend part of you that drew me to you in the first place. Honestly, though, it is hard for me to like the angry, martyr-ish side of you that I'm seeing more and more often."

"Sorry!" he shouted.

We finished getting ready and walked in silence to the dining room, where Mike warmed up. He became more attentive than usual, how's the fish, do you want to share a dessert, you look pretty tonight, etc., etc. But I was left feeling heavy and sad, wondering where we were headed.

The next afternoon, again without Mike, Bill and I sat looking out over the English Channel and talking about him. I told Bill of my frustrations and concerns, that it seemed Mike's glass was more and more often half empty. We spoke of Mike's reluctance to take care of himself—exercise, lose weight, the usual. We talked about Bill's worries for one of his sisters, how she always looked at things in the worst possible light. Bill said he had noticed more of that in Mike recently.

"Maybe we can do 'Accentuate the Positive,' tonight," Bill laughed.

"Please!"

After the walking tour, we spent a few days in London. I got sick. It gave more credibility to Mike's earlier illness, and I was left feeling guilty for thinking he just wasn't trying hard enough during the walk.

I skipped an afternoon of sightseeing. Mike brought tea up to the room on his return. For the time being at least, we were gentle with one another.

We'd been home from the England trip for three days when Mike came downstairs to tell me of an email he'd received from the pianist.

"She's quitting Yip Harburg," he said, his expression hovering somewhere between surprise and confusion.

"Quitting? Why?"

"She says it's not fun anymore."

"Really? What else did she say?"

"Just it's not fun anymore. We can't do it without her. I don't know of another pianist here in Sacramento who could do it."

"Strange," I said. "Do you mind if I read the email?"

"No. Go ahead."

I went upstairs to Mike's computer and read a very lengthy email from the pianist. She said how frustrated she'd become. They would decide on the way a particular number would go, she'd spend a week practicing, and then with the next rehearsal Mike would change everything. He would say one thing and do another. She told him how much she had always enjoyed working with him—what a fine, sensitive musician he was. She said how she had struggled with the decision, lost sleep, worried, didn't want to lose his friendship. She said she'd wanted to say all of this in person and had tried to call several times since our return, but we weren't answering our phone, nor was our answering machine taking messages. She was sorry, but the project had become overly stressful for her. It simply wasn't fun anymore.

"Not fun anymore," Mike said, shrugging his shoulders, ignoring all of the other details of her email.

Whenever Mike told others that the pianist quit, he would simply say, "She said it wasn't fun anymore."

Maybe he just didn't want to bother to explain the details of the pianist's dissatisfaction. What seems more likely to my now, though, is that he was losing, had lost, the capacity to process such details.

The bit about not answering our phones or callers being unable to leave messages was puzzling. I called our home number from a neighbor's phone. Our number rang and rang and rang. No answering machine picked up. I asked the neighbor to give me five minutes to get home, then to call me. She called, but the phone didn't ring at our place. As I thought back over the days since our return, I realized that all of our phone conversations had been with outgoing calls. When I checked with AT&T, they found that there was some glitch in which we could call out but no one could call in. I didn't know how long it had been that way, but it was certainly an added complication to uneasy communications.

The next day when we returned from running after-trip errands, the answering machine now working, there was a message from the director. She simply said she would no longer be working on the project. Mike called the others who were involved and said they would need to take a hiatus. He hoped to pick things back up again soon. Then he went upstairs to bed.

In November 2007, Mike went with me to New York for the annual Assembly on Literature for Adolescents conference. I was busy most of both days, presenting, participating in workshops, and catching up with other teachers and writers with whom I'd become acquainted over my years of attending these conferences. Mike was on his own during the day.

He had always loved New York City—the energy, the museums, the restaurants, Central Park, the big library, St. Patrick's Cathedral, the whole city. An added attraction this year was to be a meeting with Ernie Harburg, Yip's son. They'd had quite a lot of contact, both email and telephone, during planning and rehearsals of the now ill-fated show. Ernie had been enthused about the project and had been very generous in filling in information that was not easily found in books. "If you're ever in New York...." So Mike called him a few weeks before we were to leave and set up a meeting time. He was thrilled with the prospect of talking face-to-face with Ernie.

Mike was watching TV when I returned to the room after the last workshop of the day.

"How was your time with Ernie?"

"He didn't show up. We were supposed to meet in that coffee shop and he didn't show up."

He'd said the coffee shop was just across the street from his apartment, and I knew Mike had his address and phone number.

"Did you call?"

"No. He didn't show up."

"Did you go across the street and knock on his door?"

"No! He didn't show up!"

"Well, maybe you could reschedule for tomorrow. Why don't you give him a call?"

"I told you. He didn't show up!"

On the flight home as I reviewed our time in New York, I was aware of how different this trip had been from previous trips. Mike's usual pattern was to get out early for breakfast. He'd walk the streets, visit a museum, lunch in Central Park, maybe walk through Macy's, enjoy the city while I was doing conference things. Later we'd go to dinner at a place Mike had chosen, someplace quintessentially New York, respected but not totally out of our price range. Typically we'd see a show that he had arranged for. This time, though, unless I was with him, he spent most of his time in the hotel room. I'd been the one to arrange a meeting with a longtime music friend of Mike's. A workshop friend had invited us to see the Radio City Rockettes with her and her son, and we did that. But Mike had not taken the initiative for any of this.

When we returned home and people asked about our trip, Mike's response would be "Wonderful! I love that city!" He might mention the Rockettes, or meeting with his friend, but mostly it was just wonderful.

July 2013

Dear Mike,

Matt, Leesa and 8-year-old Mika flew down from Washington for a week with the California family. The evening of their arrival, Dale and Marg joined us at my place for dinner. We sat outside with martinis and some version of appetizers, talking and laughing while we waited for the River Wok delivery. Once the food arrived, we served ourselves buffet style from the kitchen and regrouped on the patio. It was a balmy Sacramento night, a light Delta breeze, and an overhead crescent moon. One of those evenings when everything seems right.

It's sometimes a challenge for me not to compare my little patio with the uneven bricks with the Gold River patios you and I had together—artfully planted, the large, sturdy glass table with plenty of comfortable places for eight people to sit. That evening we had to pull out a couple of folding chairs for our River Wok dinner. But really, my present patio served us well. The folding chairs, the smaller basic table, the funky walk down not-to-code steps and through the crowded garage to get to the patio—none of that kept us from enjoying our time together. We could still laugh and eat and drink and talk about what mattered. It turns out I don't need nearly as much as we once thought we needed together.

Dale and Marg are now party central for our larger family get-togethers. They hosted a delightful evening that, in addition to those who had been assembled on my patio, included the Stockton cousins. Later in the week Sharon and Lena and Corry joined us and, still later, Beth and Cindi. It was truly a reunion. How lucky I am to be a part of this bright, funny, varied family!

It is a delight to see Matt with Mika. He is patient and playful and, at the same time, doesn't let her get away with murder. She is full of energy and pushes a variety of boundaries, and Matt is firm without being punitive. You should be proud—you, Matt's main role model for fatherhood.

Mika has not gone to see you with Matt and Leesa these past few visits. I know you would brighten for a moment, only a moment, if you were to see her. You would not be able to interact with her. She would be left confused, watching you walk your loop. I want you to have as many bright moments as you can, no matter how brief. On the other hand, it's sad to think that her strongest image of you would be that of a demented old man. So I tend to agree with Matt and Leesa's decision to leave her with me, for ice cream and DVDs, while they make the trip to Orangevale.

When I try to think of what you might want, the old you, I think you, too, might agree with that choice. I know I would. If and when—God help us all, probably when—I become an unpleasant shell of my former self, I'd prefer that the grandkids not see me, that the memories they're left with are of the alive me, not the half-dead me. And Mika does have memories of you playing the piano and singing "Lydia the Tattooed Lady." And there's that wonderful picture of you dressed up in a long royal blue satinish robe with a very tall pointed hat, a wizard with a wand. Facing you is 3-year-old Mika in her sparkly shoes and pink princess outfit. You were both so engrossed in play that you were oblivious to the camera. Such a better memory for her than memories of a visit to you at Sister Sarah's would be.

You, the real you, are alive in that little Mika soul. When I emailed to ask what DVDs she would like me to have on hand for her visit, I listed every Disney story available, along with a variety of musicals. She chose "Singin' in the Rain." I know she watched that with you on at least one visit to Gold River. Later, on that last ill-fated visit, the one when you went missing in the Seattle airport, and again in Walla Walla, you and she sat together on the couch watching "Singin' in the Rain." You'd already lost the capacity to know your audience, and you were endlessly repeating stories of Gene Kelly and Donald O'Connor, things way beyond her 4-year-old understanding. But she watched with you for a long time, seemingly mesmerized by the singing and dancing.

That was our last visit together to Walla Walla. I can see you now, sitting at the table in the breakfast nook of that spacious Craftsman-style house they'd rented from the college. I was sitting across from you, finishing my eggs and toast. Finished with her breakfast, Mika stood at the end of the table, looking at you as if trying to figure things out. Finally she said to you, "I heard you have trouble remembering." You, who had never admitted to any such trouble to the rest of us, said, "I forget things sometimes. But I'll always remember you."

On this trip, after watching "Singing' in the Rain" for the second time, Mika asked me, "Do you have 'American in Paris?'" Somewhere within her, probably within her DNA, I believe she will also always remember you.

We will have been married for 46 years this coming Monday. The day will be like any other. Nothing to distinguish it except that memories of that long ago wedding day may push their way forward. I'll let them linger, but not for long. The contrast between *early happy memories and now is heartbreaking. It breaks my heart that we're not celebrating together. That we're not traveling, or exploring new restaurants, or having people in for dinner, or going to concerts, or sharing books or, together, watching this amazing time for Subei as she makes her way to college, or any of the other things we might reasonably have expected for our retirement years.*

On this coming anniversary, I will take a moment to honor you. To honor what we had together. And I thank you for somewhere around 38 good years. I wouldn't trade them for anything.

Still yours,
Marilyn

NOT SUCH A
MERRY CHRISTMAS

December 2007

Ever since Mike and I married in 1967, we'd hosted the family Christmases. Mike loved Christmas. The music. Decorating. Buying and wrapping presents. Making our traditional Christmas lasagna. Dale's birthday is on Christmas day, and Mike always took great pleasure in coming up with some over-the-top fancy dessert for that part of the celebration. The most memorable outrageous dessert he accomplished was the Baked Alaska of 1985. With such fancy recipes, Mike put everything together, carefully following each detailed step, and I walked around behind him, cleaning up and putting away. On that occasion, everything went as outlined in the *Gourmet* magazine recipe until he poured the ¼ cup of rum over the top and it didn't light. The next pour was more generous, and flambé it did. Mike carried the inferno to the table singing happy birthday to the ooohs and ahhhs of the gathered celebrants. I stayed in the kitchen dousing the flaming dish towel.

It was the tradition to gather at our house for Christmas Eve. Some years we did a big dinner both on Christmas Eve and on Christmas Day, but this year, 2007, we decided to make it easy on ourselves and have an early Christmas Eve dinner at a nearby restaurant before exchanging gifts back at our place.

Things took a turn at dinner when Mike asked Ashley, our 15-year-old grand-daughter, how she was liking Rio Americano High School. She said she didn't like high school and she'd shifted to independent studies through a local charter school. When Mike referred to her as a dropout, it was clear she was hurt by his remark. Mike had been totally enamored of her, and she of him in her younger days. Her teenage years were a challenge for them both, but I was surprised and saddened by the hurtfulness of Mike's accusation.

Later in the evening, presents opened, dessert served, Mike started on a rant about how any parent who would let their kid go to independent studies should have the kid removed from the home.

"Traditional high schools don't work for everyone, Mike," Jeannie said.

"Well, they should!"

He went on to say that kids shouldn't be allowed to attend alternative high schools. It was a waste of time. They didn't learn anything. And on and on. When he finished his rant, he went upstairs to bed. The rest of us sat stunned. Three of us—Dale, Jeannie and I—had taught for decades at alternative high schools. We had seen kids who had been on the verge of dropping out do some spectacular turnarounds. Small classes, more choices for study, a sense of community, close and caring guidance, worked quite well for many who had not been able to fit into the large school machine. No, they couldn't do high school sports there, or be in a chorus, or on debate team. But they got a program more in keeping with their own needs.

"How could he say that?" Jeannie asked. "How could he say that to us?"

I just shook my head. I didn't get it.

That night I did something I had only done four or five times in our whole lives together. I slept on the couch. Well, I didn't exactly sleep, but I stayed on the couch during sleep time. The few other times I had gone elsewhere to sleep, Mike had appeared after a few hours, saying something like, "Let's talk. I miss you." This was the first time he didn't come to get me, the first time I'd stayed away all night long.

Early the next morning, Mike was downstairs finishing the cleanup. I showered, then joined him. Sharon, Doug, Subei, and Lena were still sleeping. The others wouldn't arrive until early afternoon.

"Come for a walk with me," I said.

We walked in silence, a short way down the nature path that winds through Gold River and ends up at the edge of the American River. It was a beautiful, clear, sunny day.

I took Mike's hand and led him off the path. We stood under one of the many giant oak trees and I began telling him how unhappy I'd been with his behavior. I mentioned his hurtful remark to Ashley.

"Did you see the look on her face when you said that?" I asked.

I said he was positively rude to our guests, and to me, when he was so aggressively demeaning of alternative education. "It was as if you were saying our work counted for nothing."

He started in on other things, as if he'd not heard me. He was angry at the possibility that someone might bring a Coke can to the table and mar the beautiful setting he'd laid out.

"We can pour the Coke into a glass, put the can in the kitchen," I suggested.

He was angry that Cindi wouldn't help with cleanup.

"All we have to do is ask."

The more I offered solutions, the angrier Mike became. There we were, on that beautiful Christmas morning, in that beautiful setting, Mike yelling, me crying.

"Whatever happened to the kind, gentle husband I married?" I choked out.

"I'm not kind! I'm not gentle!"

"I can see that."

Eventually I said to him, "Let's just get through the day without ruining everyone else's Christmas. It's always been a fun gathering. Something we've offered to family and friends for decades. Let's not ruin it. Just for today," I asked.

A young family, boy on a tricycle, girl in a stroller, came walking by.

"Merry Christmas," the dad called out.

"Merry Christmas," the mother joined in.

"Merry Christmas!" Mike said, all light and warmth. "Beautiful day, isn't it?"

"Beautiful," the adults responded.

I was beginning to think that Dr. Jekyll and Mr. Hyde had nothing on Mike.

Dinner went smoothly, though I was constantly aware that Mike's anger was just under the surface. That became obvious as we heard news of a tragic event that had taken place at the San Francisco Zoo late Christmas afternoon. A 243-pound Siberian tiger, Tatiana, had escaped from the tiger grotto, killed one 17-year-old young man and injured two brothers, one 19 years old and the other 23. When police arrived, the 17-year-old was already dead, and the older brother was lying on the ground with cuts on his face, cornered by the tiger. The four police officers, who were yelling, caught the tiger's attention and she advanced toward them. All four fired their handguns, killing the tiger. Two witnesses said the three young men had been taunting the tiger. Not smart, or kind, but hardly worthy of a death sentence.

Dale, Mike, and I were in the kitchen, talking about what a sad event that was. The loss of the young man's life, the death of that beautiful tiger, the likely complications, legal and otherwise, it meant for the zoo.

"They shouldn't have killed that animal," Mike said.

"What could they do?" I asked. "It was coming after the officers. It was near the cafe where a few people were still at tables."

"I don't care. They shouldn't have killed her!"

"But Mike," Dale said, "what if you had been at the zoo with your grandkids and an angry tiger was on the loose?"

"They shouldn't have killed that tiger!" Mike shouted and left the room.

Later Dale asked if I thought Mike *believed* the tiger should not have been killed, or if he was just taking an opposite stance. I couldn't say. I no longer had any idea of what Mike really believed as he tossed extreme, dogmatic statements into a conversation.

Late Christmas night, with everyone gone and Mike in bed, I sat at the dining room table, thinking about the many people who had gathered around it for holiday meals and so many other less crowded dinners. Had the years of laughter and serious conversation somehow seeped into the grain of the wood? How would it be not to gather around this table at Christmastime?

The past two years of growing distance, dissatisfaction, and anger were wearing on me. I began thinking about the details of divorce or of a legal separation. Although Mike seemed to love me less, it was also apparent that he needed me more. I wondered how he would do without me. Well … he wasn't doing very well with me either. As for me, I was convinced I'd be better off without Mike's constant emotional turmoil, without the oppression of his black cloud of depression. I was banging my head against a wall, trying to make things better for Mike, and failing. Maybe it was time for me to jump out of the increasingly hot soup pot.

I looked around at our accumulation of china and crystal. Mike could have it all. He cared more about it than I ever did. I'd take the pottery set we'd chosen ages ago as we'd prepared for a life together. He could have the silver. I'd take the stainless steel.

I wandered into the living room and curled up in front of the fire on what we referred to as our "martini" couch. Newly ensconced in Gold River, back around '98 or '99, while we wandered through a furniture store in search of a small, occasional table, a big, bright, overstuffed couch caught our attention. I don't remember who moved toward it first, but we both ended up sitting on it, leaning into the supportive back, leaning into the heavily padded arms. It was unusual for us to gravitate toward the same piece of furniture. Mike usually wanted a more formal style, while I was drawn to things more casual and practical. We bought it right then. No second thoughts. No pros and cons. Who would take the couch?

The couch question moved me onto thoughts of where we each might live. Mike had come to glorify Los Angeles and to resent living in Sacramento. Perhaps he would move back to LA. I would find a much smaller place in Sacramento. But we were already living close to the financial edge. How could we afford two separate places? And how would that be for our kids and grand-kids if we split up?

We were generally compatible roommates, easily sharing household chores. Maybe that should be my relationship goal. Forget love, support, deep communication. Settle for a decent roommate. My 2008 New Year's resolution was to maintain low expectations.

The day after Christmas I told Mike we wouldn't be having it at our house the next year.

"We've always had Christmas!"

"Did you enjoy this Christmas?"

"Yes. I always enjoy Christmas!"

"It didn't seem like it. You were either angry or on the verge of anger the whole time. You were rude and inconsiderate of others. I'm not doing it with you, here, next year."

After telling the rest of the family of my decision, I called the Aliso Creek Inn in Laguna Beach and reserved three separate condominiums for December 23 through 26, 2008. Aliso Creek had long been a family favorite of ours, and it would certainly be a change of Christmas scenery. When I showed Mike the reservation, he said he wasn't going to Laguna for Christmas. He was going to have Christmas at home, just like always. I said fine, I'd miss him. But I would be in Laguna Beach.

WITHOUT A ROOM
OF ONE'S OWN
2008

Mike had for some time been directing Chanteuses, an a cappella ensemble of 16 or so women singers. He loved working with Chanteuses, all excellent singers and accomplished musicians, willing to experiment with a wide variety of pieces. He loved them, and they loved him. He would often remark that it was a joy to work with such fine singers. The Chanteuses women were equally appreciative of Mike's leadership—his capacity to bring out the best in them musically, his sensitive interpretations of a broad range of compositions, his precision, his warmth and humor.

He also sang with Camerata California, a group of professional singers and instrumentalists. Again, a group with a weekly evening rehearsal. The Yip Harburg project was stalled, probably dead. Mike was happiest when he was busy, and with his music activities now mainly consisting of only two enterprises, he was left with an abundance of time on his hands.

In early January, Mike got an email from the minister of a nearby Presbyterian church, asking if he would be interested in their newly opened position as director of choral music and, if so, might they meet within the next few days. Mike was hesitant, not wanting to again be tied down on Sundays, but I encouraged him to at least meet with the minister and give it some thought. My hope was that adding more to his music plate would have him less often in the doldrums. Also, with the downturn in the economy and my lessened book income, we sorely missed the income Mike lost when he resigned from UUSS. In January 2008, Mike started as choral director at Northminster Presbyterian church.

Although the theology was not as close to Mike's take on things religious as had been the case at UUSS, the setting was more compatible. There was a designated space for the choir in the sanctuary, a designated choir room, and choir robes—all things that had been missing at UUSS, and things that Mike considered to be important in the life of a church choir. He was welcomed warmly at

Northminster, and both choir and congregation expressed great appreciation for his talents and leadership.

During this time, Mike continued taking Cymbalta and meeting with Dr. Bertoli on a weekly basis. When he returned from a therapy session, Mike invariably said it had been a good time. He appreciated her insights. Occasionally after a session he would even say, "I think I've turned a corner." Such shifts in attitude rarely lasted for more than a few hours. He was increasingly discontent.

It was becoming more and more difficult for me to write at home. Previously respectful of my work time, Mike now came into my office whenever he felt like it. "Let's go to a movie," he'd say, or "I'm feeling depressed," or "I can't get the email to send!"

"Interrupting writing time is like interrupting a dream," I reminded him. "It's hard to get back to it once the flow is disrupted."

"I'm sorry," he might say, but it wouldn't be long before he would open the door to my office again. "Just one quick question, then I'll leave you alone."

While teaching full time, I'd managed to publish three books in a series of realistic teen fiction. Juggling writing time and teaching time, family time and time with friends was demanding and frustrating. I began toying with the idea of an early retirement. At 58, I would receive much less in retirement income than if I'd continued teaching until 62, or even 60, but I was eager to make the shift from full-time teacher/part-time writer, to full-time writer/part-time teacher. Money from royalties was gradually increasing, as was income from writing-related speaking engagements. That, coupled with a retirement plan that allowed for 30 days of school district work each year for the five years following retirement, made it seem possible. A reach, but possible.

As I was struggling with the early retirement decision, Mike and I were leading a small group of adults through *The Artist's Way* by Julia Cameron, a book devoted to nurturing and developing creativity. One of the pieces of advice that seemed appropriate to me at that time was, "Leap, and the net will appear." That spring, in 1993, I took the leap. I wasn't up for following Ms. Cameron's advice when it came to walking over bridges, but it was a useful metaphor with which to counteract my overly cautious natural tendencies. It's still a useful metaphor.

Between my retirement in 1993 and this time in 2008, I'd published five more teen novels and one nonfiction book meant for teachers, *I Won't Read and You Can't Make Me: Reaching Reluctant Teen Readers*. My general practice during those years had been to maintain a five-day work schedule—getting started sometime between 9 and 10 o'clock, after a leisurely breakfast and paper perusal with Mike, taking a lunch break near noon, then quitting sometime between 3 and 4 in the afternoon. I sometimes ignored the self-imposed regimen if the grandkids were coming over on a Friday afternoon, or if we had out-of-town visitors, or if we took a short getaway to San Francisco, or to visit the Woodacre family, but I was otherwise fairly disciplined in my work habits.

Usually I spent the morning reviewing and making changes to the previous day's writing, then completed another four or five pages that moved things along in whatever story I was working on. In the afternoons I did book/education-related business, answering email and phone calls, sometimes arranging for author visits or planning teacher workshops, though since the recession, the time needed to arrange author visits or workshops had dwindled. I made it a point not to work on weekends. But in spite of my limited and flexible work schedule, Mike became more and more resentful of any time I spent in my office.

One morning, just minutes after our leisurely breakfast time, as I was settling in to work, Mike stormed into my office and shouted angrily, "I didn't get married to live alone!"

I was generally slow to anger, but on this particular morning I snapped back.

"You so don't live alone! We have mornings together and all day after 4 o'clock. It's nothing like when you were teaching, singing regularly with the Master Chorale, doing other singing gigs and sometimes juggling a church job! Now all of a sudden you want my exclusive time and attention? Too bad! I want five to six hours a day out of 24. Weekends free. That's hardly excessive!"

A less defensive response would have been kinder, and might possibly even have been more effective. But I was worn down and, at least with Mike, had lost sight of my better self.

Another time, after a series of morning interruptions, I said, "I wouldn't think of interrupting you during a rehearsal. How can I convince you to at least wait until after lunchtime, when the creative part is done?"

"Okay!" he'd said. "I won't bother you!"

He was back within the hour. It seemed no matter how I tried to renew the idea that my work time was sacred, Mike continued to barge in whenever the impulse struck him.

For three decades of marriage I had readily adapted to Mike's busy teaching and music schedule, working around his activities to squeeze in a little piece of time with him, maybe a movie, or a dinner out, but mostly he was on the go, including Sunday mornings. It seemed totally selfish and unreasonable for him, now, to expect me to drop everything at his slightest whim. I needed a way to protect enough chunks of time to stay with my writing projects. It seemed my only choice was to take my laptop elsewhere for uninterrupted writing.

As resentful as Mike had become of my writing time, I was equally resentful of having to leave home in order to get any work done. I loved my home office, a whole wall of built-in book shelves, the 3-foot-by-6-foot tabletop desk that allowed space for several stacks of projects without feeling cluttered, the window that looked out on a giant redwood and, in season, flowering plum trees and crepe myrtles. But the only way to find uninterrupted time was to get out of the house. So I did.

Note: Unlike the other pretend letters to Mike that could never be read by him, this is an actual letter that I wrote on the stated date and planned to hand-deliver to him. However, upon re-reading what I had written, I realized the futility of expecting him to understand any of my frustrations and tucked the letter away in what was a fast-growing "Mike" file.

October 28, 2008

Dear Mike,

There is so much I want to say to you, and so little I think can get through. My life with you now is unbelievably frustrating. I would have never predicted that we would become so alienated in what had promised to be exciting, free times for us. I believe that you love me in an abstract way, but I no longer believe you love <u>me</u>. Most of the time you seem angry and withdrawn. I no longer feel that you know me, or that you even care to know me. Do you ever wonder what's going on with me, either physically or emotionally unless it's directly related to you?

I cringe at so much of what you have to say these days, your puffed up, narcissistic Leeta*-like pronouncements: "I'm never wrong!" "I hate praise music!" "I hate the guitar!" "Nothing embarrasses me!" Unlike you, I am often embarrassed by such posturing. It leaves no room for real conversation and indicates a small, closed mind. So unlike the you I once knew.

Your response to the gaffe of putting the knife and spoon on the left side of plates was to yell, "Well, they're wrong!" when you saw that the Better Homes cookbook showed the opposite. Rearranging the utensils, as if to humor me, you announced, "We can do it that way if that's what you want." In reality, I didn't care how the table was set as long as everyone had utensils with which to eat and a plate to eat from. You knew that, once.

I am so overwhelmingly weary of waking up to your litany of unhappiness. The church. Sacramento. My work. Politicians. Neighbors. At 7 o'clock in the morning, that martyred sigh, "I have such a long day today …" It's hard for me to sympathize when you've got a whole day before you until 4 o'clock, 3:30 if we count drive time. And then you'll be back by 9:30 or 10 o'clock? Hardly like those earlier days when you were often out of the house by 6 in the morning, and not home until 11.

I am caught in an ever tightening vice. Whatever I try to talk with you about elicits some kind of knee-jerk response—you don't get me, or nobody can tell me what to do, or … whatever. I'm left without a voice.

You're resentful of your life being "monitored." As distant as we are from one another now, I am still greatly concerned for your well-being. It is disheartening to me that you've let yourself go physically. You who have so carefully nurtured your God-given musical talent and voice, are squandering your God-given strong, healthy body. Your diet is atrocious, and you've tipped the scale to obesity.

Enough for now. I have so little hope for us, and every time I allow for hope, it all vaporizes into thin air.

Ever so sincerely,
Marilyn

*Leeta was Mike's very difficult mother—narcissistic long before it was ever designated as a personality disorder by the Diagnostic and Statistical Manual of Mental Disorders.

I DON'T KNOW
WHERE YOU ARE
2008

The middle school librarian who had successfully fought the strongest challenge of the 2006 challenges that put *Detour for Emmy* on that year's top 10 banned books list received the 2007 Texas Library Association Intellectual Freedom Award. Although she was definitely the one on the front lines of the censorship battle, I had helped with backup information and an op-ed for their local newspaper. As a result, the two of us were invited to speak at several library association conferences, one of which was the 2008 Texas School Library Association gathering in Dallas.

I checked the map and found that while in Dallas, I would be a mere 230 miles from Macedonia, Arkansas, the place where my father and his 10 brothers and sisters grew up.

I called Dale. "I don't think I can be so close to Macedonia and not drop by. Wanna do a road trip?"

A week before the conference, Dale and I flew to Dallas, rented a car, and made the pilgrimage to Macedonia. Well ... we actually headed for Magnolia, the town a few miles north of Macedonia that had a motel and several little cafes.

We had a long history of such pilgrimages. During the time of our growing up, our father allowed himself the luxury of a vacation every four years, and we would make the road trip from Temple City, California, to Macedonia, Arkansas.

Although Dale and I didn't see our Arkansas relatives often, we were nevertheless closely connected. As adults we continued the visits, though the timing wasn't as predictable as the old four-year cycle.

By this time, all of our father's laughing, storytelling, salt-of-the-earth brothers and sisters were gone, as was he. Most of our cousins now lived elsewhere. But our 90-year-old cousin, Pauline, was still alive and in her house in Macedonia. We decided it was best not to tell Pauline we were coming. She was wheelchair-bound, but we knew she would want us to stay with her. We also knew she would have been undone by not being able to offer the level of hospitality that would live up to her standards.

Other than Pauline, we weren't sure who else we might see.

We spent the night in Dallas and called a cousin, Billy Wayne, who lived in Longview, to say we would be traveling through and did he want to meet for lunch. He told us he'd meet us at a Waffle House just off the I-20 and gave directions complete with the freeway exit number and plenty of landmarks. Had it been 20 years since we'd seen him? More? We took up where we left off.

He'd retired from Eastman when they expected him to start using a computer. He loved retirement the first few years, but then his wife, Beth, retired from her work as a school librarian.

"I could hardly stand that! I guess she couldn't either 'cause she went back to work six months after she retired."

"How much longer will she work?" I asked.

"'Til one of us drops dead, I hope."

Once settled in our motel rooms in Magnolia, it was with some trepidation that Dale called Pauline. Would she be alert? Would she remember us? She answered the phone. "Where are you?? Get yourself on down here," she told him, laughing her raucous, distinctive laugh.

We were welcomed by cousins we'd not seen in decades. David, the cousin we'd kept in closest contact with over the years, was just two years younger than I. We'd not seen each other often as kids, but when we did, we were immediate good buddies. He and his stepbrother, someone we'd also been quite fond of, drove down from Monticello, Arkansas, to see us. We all gathered at Pauline's one afternoon. She told story after story, some we'd heard over the years and some with pieces of new information. It was a magical time.

I emailed Mike with pictures from our gathering at Pauline's, telling him how lucky I felt to be reconnecting, and how easily things had come together. When I talked with him the next evening, he only wanted to know when I was coming home.

"Did you get my email with the pictures?"

"Yes," he said, but he had nothing to say about them, or my account of our time with Pauline. Mike had visited Pauline on two different trips. When we were there in 1994, he'd been so impressed with her tomato "piccalilli" that he'd watched carefully while she put a batch together, writing down approximate amounts of ingredients and the steps to completion. It looked so easy when Pauline was doing it, sitting in her chair in the living room, cutting up tomatoes and onions and various other vegetables, dropping the pieces into a big pan that sat on her footstool. When the pan was full, she carried it to the stove, turned the fire on under it, and soon we had that wonderful relish.

We'd determined to make some when we got home. It took us most of one full day to gather the ingredients, cut them up, and cook them. We ended up with three puny jars. Mike's take on it was that only Pauline could be Pauline. They'd connected on both of Mike's visits, and he was one of the first people she asked about when we got to her place that April. But Mike seemed indifferent to anything I had to tell him about her—eager for me to finish the story so he could ask when I was coming home.

Every phone call between us started and ended with Mike asking, "When are you coming home?" I would again tell him the date. I'd remind him that my return flight information was written on the calendar and also that he had my itinerary in his email. But the next conversation would be the same. Once he'd called in the middle of the afternoon. When I picked up, he didn't even bother to say hello, just, angrily, "When are you coming home?"

In contrast, Marg was soaking up every detail of Dale's emails and phone calls. She could not have been happier for us—how happy she was that we were reconnecting with these dear people. How lucky for Dale and me to have this time together, etc. I wanted some of that same enthusiasm from Mike, but what I know now that I didn't know then was that he had already lost the capacity to resonate with anyone else's emotions or experiences.

Once I got back home, Jeannie told me of a strange experience she'd had with Mike. They'd met for lunch, as they did fairly often. Over lunch Mike had told Jeannie, "I have no idea where Marilyn is."

She was taken aback.

"I know where she is," she'd said. "She's with Dale in Arkansas, visiting family."

A little later over lunch he'd made the same remark. "I have no idea where Marilyn is."

When our Arkansas visit was over, we drove back to Dallas where Dale caught a flight back to Sacramento, and I went on to the conference. It was a great success, fun and, according to participants, informative regarding ways to meet book challenges. But Mike was as indifferent to talk of my conference experiences as he had been to my Arkansas experiences. I took it as further evidence that he had simply ceased to care about me.

Looking back, I see that dealing with email had already become difficult for Mike. I now doubt that he'd even read the emails or seen the pictures I'd sent. I also think he may *truly* not have known where I was. And he may not have known from one day to the next when I was coming home. No wonder he was distraught! But all I knew then was that I was less and less able to reach him in any meaningful way. And yet, there were still rare times that gave me hope. Times that kept me from jumping out of the soup pot. A case in point was Northminster Presbyterian's summer choir picnic, held in the welcoming and spacious backyard of one of the choir members.

Mike did what he had always done at the end of a choir season, whether with high school singers, church singers, or other choral groups. He gave awards and tributes to each of the singers. No one was left out, and none of it was phony. He had an uncanny knack for finding the best in each choir member and honoring that. He made the presentations with grace and gentle humor, but never humor in the slightest way at anyone's expense. On their part, members of the choir and other church staff heaped accolades on Mike—his warmth and musicianship, his capacity for bringing out the highest quality of music they were able to produce. It was a love fest on all sides and a welcome three hours when the old Mike was on the scene.

On that day, as on so many past days, he'd made it a point to include me in conversations, connect me with other teachers there, occasionally mention my books. When we left, I allowed myself to hope. Maybe the therapy was working after all. Maybe the meds were kicking in. Maybe. Maybe. Maybe.

"THERE'S NOTHING WRONG WITH ME!"

June 2008

Our adult kids noticed that we had become easily irritated with one another, but attributed it to a change in our relationship. I did, too, at first. Something was wrong between us that I couldn't understand or fix, and after 40 years together I was seriously considering separation if not divorce. But I'd also begun to think that maybe there was more to Mike's changes than trouble in our relationship could explain.

At first when I would express my concerns to friends, they might remind me of Mike's "artist's personality," or even scoff, saying he was the same good-time Mike they'd always known. Closest family and friends, though, were beginning to note some puzzling observations of their own. Dale remarked that when he and another good friend, Dave, met for their regular monthly lunches, Mike no longer took much of an interest in what either he or Dave was saying. However, he was still quite interested in what *he* had to say, at times getting stuck on one subject to the exclusion of all else.

On a weekend visit, Sharon mentioned that it was painful watching Mike try to make pie dough. One of his areas of expertise had been pies, always making a pecan pie and a pumpkin pie, both from scratch, for our Thanksgiving dinners. Then one day he got the pie dough wrong. That can happen to anyone. Even Julia Child made mistakes in the kitchen. But it was notable.

Other ominous signs were emerging. Mike had always kept our social calendar. We checked dates with one another, but he was the busiest, performing as a singer, or organizing and conducting concerts, so the master calendar task fell to him. Then gradually, without at first even being fully conscious of the change, I was more and more checking dates. Then I noticed that people who had arranged a date with Mike might also email me to confirm that date. Changes in Mike began to be a major topic of family conversation. What was going on?

In June we joined family and friends in Woodacre for Sharon's 50th birthday party. Although she was not Mike's daughter from birth, he loved her as if she were. And she, at the age of 9, had finally gotten the kind of dad she'd always wanted.

Shortly after we married in 1967, Mike adopted Sharon and Cindi, happily and wholeheartedly becoming their father. Two years later, when Sharon was 10½ and Cindi had just turned 9, our son, Matt, was born. We all doted on him, to the point of arguing over who got to give him his evening bath. We were a family of five, not counting pets.

At the Woodacre party, Mike raised his glass to toast Sharon's 50th birthday. He talked of his respect for her and for her dedication to education. He spoke of her work at Sonoma State College, and of her great achievement in becoming a Doctor of Chiropractic. And then he took a turn, saying that, of course, he hadn't been at her high school graduation because he was still living in Tampa at the time.

In truth, he'd not lived in Tampa since he'd left home for college in 1958.

I laughed and said, "We were all living together in Altadena then."

He turned to me, angry, and said, "No, I wasn't! I was in Tampa when Sharon graduated from high school!"

For the people who didn't know our history, who were most of the people at the party, either version sounded credible. But the 10 or so people who did know our history stood looking wide-eyed and puzzled. Though in truth Mike never drank to excess, Jeannie made a joke of taking Mike's wine glass from him.

"No more for you," she said.

The tension eased, someone else made a toast, and the party continued.

Later, when only family was left and Mike had gone to bed, several of us sat outside on the deck, talking about Mike's time gaffe, and also citing other puzzling incidents we'd noticed over the past year or so. It was no longer "things aren't right between Mom and Dad," it was "what's going on with Mike/Dad?"

Sharon, the holistic medicine chiropractor, said that if it were Doug, she would get him off of all drugs. Marg, an RN, thought that might not make a big difference, though she said sometimes the immediate cessation could bring improvement for a short period of time, then the difficulties that were being treated by meds would often return with more intensity. I was having a hard enough time dealing with Mike. To take it upon myself to start experimenting with his meds seemed risky to me.

When we awakened the morning after Sharon's party, I said, "You don't really think you were in Tampa when Sharon graduated from high school, do you?"

"I was in Tampa," Mike insisted.

I tried to walk him back through the time of our marriage, Sharon and Cindi's participation in his children's church choir, his taking Sharon to piano lessons when she was in the ninth grade, but he would have none of it.

"I don't like it when you contradict me!" he said.

"Then stop making such ridiculous statements!"

On the way home I told Mike how concerned I was about him. I cited missed appointments and other time gaffes. I urged him to see our doctor. He resisted.

"There's nothing wrong with me!" he said, then closed his eyes and went to sleep.

June 2013

Dear Mike,

I'm sitting at the big glass table in Jerry and Jackie's* condominium at Madeira Beach. How strange it is to be in Florida without you—to wake in the mornings, in the bed we shared on past trips and watch, alone, the giant pelicans fly close past the eighth-story balcony. Last night I slept with the drapes drawn and the sliders open. I don't think any of the Florida family ever do that, but how we loved being lulled to sleep by the gentle rhythm of the gulf waves. I continue the now lonely tradition.

Beth** stayed over last night. We had wine and cheese on the balcony and talked until we could hardly keep our eyes open. Before the rest of the Baptists return later in the week, we'll dispose of the evidence of our sins.

Much of the talk was of you, Mike. You hold such a warm, favorite-uncle place in Beth's heart. When you and I were down here in 2009, just after you'd been diagnosed with frontotemporal dementia, Beth was frantic to find a treatment, or something to stop the progression. She followed the path the rest of us, Doug, Sharon, Matt, Dale, Marg, and I had followed earlier on. Sadly, her search was as futile as ours had been. She now, like so many other close friends and family, has become numbed to the reality that the essence of you is gone from us, and it's not coming back. You are sorely missed. Not a day, not an hour, goes by that I don't think of you, and even when the frequency of such thoughts dwindles, I know it: I will never fully stop missing you.

Joan Kaywell was the impetus for this Florida visit. A few years back she asked that I donate my "papers" to the Ted Hipple Memorial Special Collection at the University of South Florida. I told her everything was in total disarray, and I wouldn't know where to start. "Dump it all in a box and mail it to us. Let the librarians sort through it," she said. But as much as I wanted to continue the task of clearing things out, finding the boxes of writing related papers in Joe and Kathy's barn, and in my garage, and repacking them for mailing, was not high on my list of priorities.

Because Morning Glory Press no longer sends me to English teachers' conferences, Joan and I haven't seen much of each other these past few years, but we reconnected when she emailed, asking for a signed hardcover copy of Too Soon for Jeff *for the collection. I sent one off. She called to thank me. In the course of our conversation we allowed as how we'd been missing each other. She invited me back for a visit, suggesting*

I bring a suitcase full of my papers. I confessed that my present travel budget would get me as far as south Sacramento. Within an hour, she and Frank called and said they wanted to bring me back using their rewards miles. I was surprised and touched by their generosity and accepted their offer without hesitation.

The old me, the me you knew back when we were solvent, would have been loathe to accept such a gift—concerned about putting someone out, or exploiting a friendship, or even about not wanting to be left with a sense of obligation. But back when I was most in need, in the midst of caring for you, and later during those months without a home base, and living with the loss of so much that had been ours together, I learned to welcome the support of others with gratitude.

I landed in Tampa last Tuesday a little after 1 o'clock in the morning, the plane having been delayed for hours in Dallas/Fort Worth. Joan was waiting for me at baggage claim, all smiles in spite of the late hour. I easily grabbed the red suitcase from the carousel—the suitcase that had gone with us to England, Akumal, and Italy, plenty of other less exotic travels. Then with all the strength I could muster, I dragged your suitcase off. It was crammed with books, letters and manuscripts, and barely squeezed under the maximum weight allowance when it was checked in Sacramento.

When we got back to their house, Frank was waiting with an opened bottle of wine and an offer of snacks. I'd already eaten during the long layover, but as you know, I'm not one to turn down an offer of wine. We stayed up until after 3 o'clock in the morning. Poor Joan had to work the next day, though she didn't have to go in until 11 or so. Still, a short night for her, but we had much to get caught up with.

As is so often true, especially with people I've not seen for a while, we spoke of you at length, the tragedy of your loss of cognition, the randomness of life. Joan and Frank have a list of people for whom they pray every morning, and we are both included on that list. Jerry and Jackie, too, pray for us every day. Although such prayers are not my own practice, I appreciate the kindness of their daily remembrances.

Now 5:30 in the evening, after a sunny, clear day, the sky turns grey and within moments there is the boom of thunder. Soon a flash of lightning, more thunder, and I wonder if we're going to get one of those electrical storms I've learned to expect while in Florida. Oh, yay! Another bright flash of lightning and the crack of thunder within a millisecond!

Where was I? Joan and Frank. They are very happy together, and hospitable. Who could have predicted? Frank sometimes refers to Joan as his lesbian wife. For one who had never been in a sexual relationship with a man until Frank, now in her mid-50s, she's apparently made an easy transition. While Joan dragged herself off to work and Frank did what he does around the house, I had a long soak in their whirlpool—just what I needed after spending much of yesterday crammed into totally filled airplanes with seats that could comfortably hold most 7-year-olds.

Thursday we hauled the suitcase of papers to the University of South Florida Education building where the Hipple Collection is housed. They are mainly interested in anything pertaining to YA fiction, so after they have a chance to go through it all, the adult books and manuscripts will be sent back to me. The truth is that although talking about my "papers" seems overblown, I feel honored to have my work included in the collection.

In the afternoon, Beth picked me up at USF and took me to Jerry and Jackie's. That evening the whole Tampa family came over for dinner—Larry, Laura and Ryan, Beth, Paul, Lindsay and Laura. Maggie was away at summer camp but will be back tomorrow. David will also be in town for a few days, so by the end of the visit I will have seen all of Jerry and Jackie's kids and grandkids except for Laura and Larry's son, Stephen, who is in Geneva on an internship.

For dinner, Jerry brought in an abundance of Cuban sandwiches, yellow rice and beans—how you would have loved that.

As I prepared for this trip, memories of our first trip to Florida to visit your family kept rising to the surface. It was 1967. You, me, Sharon and Cindi—our "honeymoon." Thank you for being a father to those two little girls—now both in their 50s. Yikes!

I'm on my way to the rocker on the balcony—a little wine and cheese while I watch the sunset. Not nearly the same without you, but the sunset is still worth watching.

Thinking of you morning and night.
Marilyn

*Mike's brother and sister-in-law
** Jerry and Jackie's daughter, Mike's niece

AN ILLUSION OF
NORMALITY

July through December 2008

In spite of growing concerns and attempts to make sense of what was happening with Mike, there remained a semblance of normality in our daily lives. We were both thrilled with the election of Barack Obama, feeling for the first time since our country's invasion of Iraq that there was a possibility we might have the patient leadership necessary to work more through diplomacy than through war. We were together in our hope that our new president would be someone who could deal with complexity rather than offering simple answers.

Mike continued to be the jovial grandpa, taking the kids to our community pool and swimming with them, then providing sugary snacks of the sort they didn't often get at home.

Dinners and movies with friends, overnight visits from SoCal pals, a few days with family at Stinson Beach, breakfasts at the Gold Miner, the trappings of our lives were in place.

In early July, Mike flew to Denver where he met Matt, who was on his way from Pittsburg to Washington state, driving a U-Haul full of his, Leesa's and Mika's accumulated possessions. After having completed his Ph.D. three years earlier, Matt had been employed from year to year in positions that were prestigious, but not ongoing. Now he was starting a tenure-track position at Whitman College, a small liberal arts college in Walla Walla, Washington. It was exciting and a relief for him to be launched on a career path in a position that would be steady, challenging and meaningful. But the cross-country move was a task of mammoth proportions, and Mike was eager to help.

The two of them, Mike and Matt, shared the driving from Denver on. Leesa and 2-year-old Mika met them in Walla Walla the day after they'd arrived. Mike stayed on a few more days to help them get settled. He came home happy about his time with Matt, enthused about the town of Walla Walla, the beauty of the Whitman College campus, the house "the kids" had moved into, and, above all, the brilliance and beauty of little Mika.

Although Matt was appreciative of Mike's help, his take on their time together was not quite so glowing. One morning shortly after Mike returned home, Matt sent a gentle, loving email, outlining some of his observations and concerns:

July 11, 2008
Dear Dad,

Now that we've arrived and settled down a bit, I wanted to thank you so much for joining me on the final leg of a tough trip.... I was anticipating a relaxing time in Denver and a nice, easy drive the rest of the way to Sacramento. As it panned out, I felt too stressed and distracted to enjoy much of the trip, and I'm sorry if I wasn't very good company. I was hoping for something more along the lines of our time in LA six years ago (six!!) when you helped me find an apartment. It has meant so much to have your help and encouragement, to feel your excitement and enthusiasm during these major life-changing markers. Your love, friendship and unconditional support are precious to me, and I am continually grateful for who you are and the father you have been to me.

We talked last week and during the trip about how you're feeling these days. You said to me in the car that you were willing to look at anything about yourself—another trait that I know to be true. Your capacity for self-reflection is something else that is very important to me, something that I've learned from and tried to emulate in my own life. Well ... now the tough part. As I mentioned, I was concerned because you seem to be repeating yourself and losing your train of thought more frequently. You said that Mom had raised the same issue with you. There were a few things I noticed in particular that may be minor but are also uncharacteristic of how I've known you to act. You seemed to get disoriented in the hotel lobby whenever we stepped out of the elevator. In general, you seem more easily distracted. And, not to harp on this, but it was difficult to follow your speech at Sharon's party—a kind of tic or slip I've noticed on other occasions as well. To describe the phenomenon more specifically, it's almost as if you're inserting non-sequiturs into a conversation. For those who know you it's fairly simple to follow, but there have been times I've noticed slightly confused looks on the faces of those less familiar with your history.

I've since talked to Mom a bit more about this, and, as you know, she's very concerned. It's clear she feels a sense of urgency, and she's indicated that you seem hesitant to look closely at this issue—at times, even a bit defensive about it. She and I discussed some possible factors, including the general dynamics of your relationship with each other, depression, your medications and the issue of "living in your head" (something I can completely identify with). And, of course, we wondered if there might be something physiological going on. This last possibility is scary to us, as I know it would be and is to you. Because these kinds of issues are both terrifying and a fact of life for anyone who lives long enough, I wanted to encourage you to get some kind of professional evaluation. I have a strong feeling that these tics or mental hiccups or distracted interactions (whatever they should be called) have multiple causes, one of which MAY be physical. But a doctor's assessment would help put to rest many of Mom's (and my) concerns.

This is a hard email to write, Dad, and I'm sorry to collapse these two issues into each other in this message—the one so positive and the other so difficult. But they are not unrelated, and if something physical is going on with you, it's really important to address it as soon as possible. As I said the other day, I love you so much, and now that Mika, this amazing new person, has been added to our lives, I want to make sure you're present on this earth for as long as possible. (Not that I didn't want that before, too.) I guess in that way I'm hoping you will consider getting an evaluation not just for Mom but for me and for Mika and for the considerably large group of people who love you and selfishly want the same things.

Please let me know what you think.—Matt

Mike responded:

Dear Matt,

Thank you for the honesty of this email. I know it was not easy to write.

I continue to believe that there is nothing physically going on in my head or body, but have not ruled out that possibility. I have a physical coming up soon, and will discuss this with my doctor.

I continue to think that I've put myself in the wrong place when deciding to leave LA. Sacramento just doesn't offer enough to satisfy me emotionally or musically. I wish that this were not the case, primarily because Mom is quite happy here. I tend to live a great deal in my head, and that gets me in trouble with myself and with other family members. I often have a strong need to distance myself from the "noise" and the chaos of the house. I really meant to share with you the book about the Highly Sensitive Person. I think sometimes that I've put myself between a rock and a hard place. I care deeply for this family and for what we stand for, but find too often that I have a strong need to keep some distance for my own sake/safety/sanity. I have all too often found this a great burden, and wish that it were otherwise.

I often hunger for Intellegical [sic] involvement, and know that I've put myself, knowingly in a church that is not going to offer that. Once again I've perhaps sabotaged myself unwittingly. I only know how to put one foot in front of the other. I think I learned that at a very early age from a most unknowing, uninvolved mother.

I know that you know how very proud I am of you and Leesa and Mika. I continue to believe that it is not possible to love you more deeply. I look forward to the trip to Walla Walla and the visit with all three of you.

Thank you again for taking the time and energy to write these thoughts. I have printed them out and will re-read them again as I continue to "digest" them over the next few days.

Give Mika a big kiss from Grampa.

I love you all.
Dad

As with his perception of the pianist's detailed explanation of why she could no longer work on the Yip Harburg program, Mike seemed not to take in many of the details of Matt's message. He was touched by Matt's tributes to him in the first paragraph but rather than addressing Matt's specific concerns, he went to his now fallback position that there was nothing wrong with his head, and to an accounting of dissatisfactions with his half-empty life. Though his complaints about Sacramento and the church had become like a broken record to me, parts of his response were more puzzling. I didn't understand what he meant by "the 'noise' and the chaos of the house." I didn't understand how living in his head got him in trouble with family members. And what did he mean by "this family" as if he were not a part of it? But Mike and I had become so distanced and defensive with one another that I didn't even try to talk with him about any of that.

In September, we enjoyed an overnight in San Francisco. We walked from the Inn at the Opera to Davies Symphony Hall, where we both thoroughly enjoyed selections from Mozart and Tchaikovsky conducted by Michael Tilson Thomas. The evening was brisk but pleasant, and after the performance we walked to Jardinière, where we sipped Kahlua and cream and relived moments from the concert, including the overly friendly woman who sat on Mike's other side and at one point rested her head on his shoulder.

"I should have kicked her butt!" I told him.

"She outweighed you," he said, which is, of course, the perfect thing for any man to say to his unsuccessfully dieting wife.

The next morning we wandered through Golden Gate Park, then went to the de Young where we browsed through the textile collection, looked at the American Sculpture and Decorative Art galleries and then ate soup and salad in the cafe before heading back home.

Mike loved the San Francisco Symphony, the de Young, our little hotel, breakfast at Sears, ambling through Macy's, the city of San Francisco. All of it. He was at his best in this setting. For that very brief period it seemed that all was well. Maybe it was. Maybe it could be.

In the fall the Northminster choir work resumed, as did rehearsals for Chanteuses and Camerata. I began asking Mike for the Christmas choir schedule so we could figure out how to work around that for our Laguna Beach Christmas getaway, but Mike continued to say we were having Christmas at home, and no schedule was forthcoming.

When Mike still had not provided a choir schedule by early November, I emailed the choir president, telling her I was juggling dates for family gatherings, and asking that she send me a copy of their December schedule. She quickly complied. The only conflict in the Laguna Beach/choir dates was for the Christmas Eve concert. I made a reservation on Southwest for Mike to fly back to Sacramento on the afternoon of Christmas Eve day, and to return to Orange County airport on Christmas morning. I went over all of the plans with Mike. He reiterated that he was staying home for Christmas.

"Okay," I said, and put the flight reservation information and receipt in the Laguna/Christmas folder.

WILD GOOSE CHASES

Fall 2008

A month or so after Mike's help with Matt and Leesa's move to Walla Walla, with strong encouragement from both Matt and Sharon, Mike agreed to see Dr. Carlson, our primary care provider, for a complete evaluation. I made the appointment and, with his permission, went with him.

Mike told Dr. Carlson he didn't think there was anything wrong with him; he'd just come because the kids and I wanted him to. To begin with, Dr. Carlson asked Mike a series of questions. Was he having trouble keeping track of dates? No, he kept everything in his datebook. Trouble organizing things? No, she should see his sock drawer. Did he snore? "Marilyn says I do, but I don't think so." Was he ever aware of irregular breathing coupled with snoring? Never. Did he ever become lost when he was away from home? No. How was the therapy going with Dr. Bertoli? Great! He loved her! Did he think it was helping with the depression? Yes, she was very helpful.

Then it was my turn. I mentioned the time he left a movie in El Dorado Hills and got all the way to Pollock Pines, 40 miles from home, before he realized he'd been going in the wrong direction. I told of the strange incident at Sharon's birthday when Mike insisted he'd been living in Tampa at the time of her high school graduation, rather than having lived with her, as her dad, from the time she was 9 years old. That strange misperception had been the catalyst for having him checked out. I said he often snored, snorted, sometimes gasped for air in his sleep. He missed appointments. Some bills he paid twice, others he left unpaid. He nearly constantly reported that he was depressed, or feeling discouraged. He often complained of feeling unwell, and of headaches, nothing he'd ever been prone to in the past. Unless he had specific plans for a day, he often went back to bed around 10 in the morning, something that would have been highly unusual even just a year or so earlier. He sometimes said bed was the only place he felt safe.

Dr. Carlson ordered a number of evaluations—a neuropsychological examination, an MRI, a sleep apnea assessment at a local sleep clinic, the usual lab tests. The neuropsychological exam was set for August 18, 2008. Unsure whether or not Mike could find the office, I drove him to that appointment. When we pulled into the parking lot, Mike said he wasn't going in. He didn't want an MRI. There was nothing wrong with his brain.

"This isn't for an MRI," I told him. "That's not for another two weeks. This is the neuropsychologist. Remember? Dr. Carlson set it up. He's a psychologist who'll do an evaluation, then get it to Dr. Carlson."

"I'm not going!" he said.

"Let's just check it out," I said, getting out of the car.

Mike sat rigid in the passenger seat. I walked to his side of the car and opened the door.

"Let's just go meet this person. We have an appointment."

Mike reluctantly followed me into the office. Dr. Parker came to the lobby to greet us just moments after we sat down. He said he'd like to see Mike first, then, if we agreed, he'd like to talk with the two of us together near the end of the session. We both said that was fine. Mike fell back into his sociable default mode and cheerfully followed Dr. Parker to the examining room.

I browsed through an issue of *Psychology Today*, pausing briefly at an article on the seeming miraculous powers of blueberries to fight the ravages of time in both brain and body. I made a mental note to add blueberries to my shopping list—wild, organic blueberries. A short article in a months-old *Time* magazine left me with a sliver of hope that we might soon have a bright, articulate, reasonable person in the White House.

After half an hour or so, Dr. Parker called me back to his office. He asked a few basic questions about my life and history, then asked about my specific concerns for Mike. I kept it short, not wanting to bombard Mike with a long list of all that was going wrong. He was defensive enough as it was. I mentioned Mike's growing difficulties in keeping track of appointments, his inability to respond to email without help, and his recent problems with using the ATM.

Dr. Parker advised that Mike come in for a series of three sessions for the stated purposes of ruling out the possibilities of dementia, substance induced memory deficits, and/or AD/HD (attention deficit/hyperactivity disorder).

"Sound okay?" Dr. Parker asked.

"Sure," Mike said, smiling.

When we got to the car Mike said, "I'm not going back there!"

"Really?"

"It's just a wild goose chase. There's nothing wrong with my brain!"

"You seemed to like him."

"He wanted to play cards!" Mike said angrily. "I was raised Southern Baptist. We weren't allowed to play cards!"

As part of that first day's evaluation, Dr. Parker had apparently used a deck of common playing cards to set up a game of concentration. It was puzzling to me that Mike, who had run fast and far from the Southern Baptist fundamentalism he'd grown up with, would be offended by a deck of cards. But he was definitely offended. I turned the conversation to one of the few easy topics still in our repertoire—dinner.

Later that evening, Matt called Mike to see how the appointment had gone.

"He just wanted to play cards! It's a wild goose chase!"

Playing cards became the theme whenever he spoke of those sessions. I sat in on parts of each session and saw that Mike's social skills made him appear to be more competent than many of his everyday actions would indicate. The stories he told sounded credible. He mentioned to Dr. Parker that he would get a song stuck in his head, and he'd have to get up in the middle of the night, go downstairs and play it on the piano to get rid of it. I didn't doubt that he would get a song stuck in his head—doesn't everyone? But he never once got up in the middle of the night and went downstairs to play the piano. Still, it seemed petty and disrespectful to sit in that office and contradict the details for much of what Mike was saying. And any disagreement of fact raised his hackles. So unless it was a crucial piece of information—say, what meds he was on, or how much exercise was he getting—I let a lot slide by. As to the story about getting up out of bed and going downstairs to play the piano and other equally untrue but harmless stories that crept into Mike's conversations, I later learned there was a name for such behavior in the dementia nomenclature—confabulations—and that they were a symptom of certain aspects of dementia. But that knowledge was yet to come, along with so many other pieces of disheartening information.

After three sessions, Mike and I met with Dr. Parker to go over the results of various tests and talk about his evaluations. He said that because Mike was right-brain creative, and because his scored profile was so odd, it was difficult to achieve a definite diagnosis. Although the combined tests generally showed that there was some cognitive impairment, his memory loss did not fit a pre-Alzheimer's pattern. That was a huge relief to me! I would not have been so relieved had I known then what lay ahead.

On the basic tests Mike scored well for general information and jigsaw puzzle, low for math and very low in searching visually for images. The last score surprised me because Mike's absorption of visual information was always so much greater than mine. I remember a conversation driving home from a party many years ago that went something like this:

"Did you talk with the woman just here from Minnesota?"

"The blond, in the green dress?"

"She has a daughter at Alhambra High School."

"Big dangly earrings?"

"She wants to get her California Teaching Credential."

"Fake pearls?"

An extreme but not terribly rare example that emphasized the differences in the dominant senses through which we perceived the world. I took in the words but likely couldn't say what color the room was in which they were spoken. Mike could give every detail of appearances though not so much of conversation. The whole thing amused us, and we often relied on one another to fill in the blanks.

When I expressed my surprise that Mike scored low in the visual image category, Dr. Parker said that could be an indicator of possible ADD. Low math skills also pointed to the possibility of ADD as a child.

A few days after our visit to Dr. Parker, when I was in Dr. Bertoli 's lobby, waiting for Mike to finish his weekly therapy session, I came upon an attention-grabbing article in *Science* magazine. It was by Dr. Duane Graveline, a physician and former astronaut, and linked Lipitor and memory loss—Lipitor, which Mike had been taking for decades to combat his genetic propensity toward very high cholesterol levels. Dr. Graveline relayed a compelling story of temporarily losing much of his short-term memory after being given Lipitor to lower his cholesterol. That problem ceased shortly after he stopped taking the drug. A year later, because of ongoing elevated cholesterol readings, he agreed to resume the drug at half-dose. Soon after that, he again lost short-term memory and was diagnosed with Transient Global Amnesia, a condition that erases recall of recent events and that put Dr. Graveline back to his 13-year-old self. He didn't recognize his wife and found it amusing that anyone would think he was married with children. He wrote of his slow recovery, a combination of avoiding statins and taking various supplements, and of his ongoing research regarding statin drugs and their myriad of side effects, including some that were extremely damaging to the brain.

When Dr. Bertoli walked out with Mike, I told them of what I'd just read and asked to borrow the magazine. Back home, I rushed to my computer and did what any concerned wife would do: I searched the net for links to statins and cognitive function, finding report after report of similar experiences. Mike didn't seem to absorb much of the information I tried to pass on to him, but he did say he'd be willing to stop taking Lipitor. When Dr. Carlson returned my call later that afternoon, she was doubtful that Lipitor was the culprit, but agreed to switch Mike to a non-statin cholesterol-lowering drug.

Dr. Parker repeated tests a few weeks after Mike stopped taking Lipitor. He showed some improvement. Could it be that simple? No. Nothing was simple. But I was grasping at some cause that could be addressed, that could make things better. Whatever slight improvement Mike showed was, I now think, accidental. At the time it gave one of those not infrequent, short-lived glimmers of hope.

In Dr. Parker's "Summary and Conclusions" of the three sessions of testing, observation, and conversation with Mike, he stated that Mike showed impairment in Working Memory and Processing Speed, and that he also exhibited "symptoms of chronic undiagnosed AD/HD, complicated now by depression, medication side effects and aging." He ruled out bipolar disorder and, on the basis of other tests, concluded that Mike was "an intelligent, artistic and capable individual … able to compensate at times for his extreme distractibility and inattention…. He allowed as how Mike was unable to fully compensate in all circumstances.

The brochures available in Dr. Parker's waiting room offered information on the symptoms and possible treatments of AD/HD/ADD, and where to find support groups for both adults and children. He gave Mike a lengthy AD/HD checklist that included sections related to inattention/distractibility, impulsivity, activity level problems (both over activity and underactivity), noncompliance, underachievement/disorganization/learning problems, emotional difficulties, poor peer relations, and impaired family relationships. Mike gave it a quick glance and left it untouched on the kitchen counter. That would have given him a check in the "very much" category of "short attention span, especially for low-interest activities." On the other hand, couldn't about 99 percent of the population check that box?

Although I was aware of Dr. Parker's bias toward AD/HD, I was willing to cling to any possible diagnosis that offered a specific treatment. Dr. Parker's suggestions for treatment included a review of meds and a recommendation that Mike stop taking Topamax, which he said sometimes had memory loss side effects. He recommended that Mike take Ritalin to address possible AD/HD. He suggested starting Aricept, often used with Alzheimer's but also with other age-related cognitive impairment. He also recommended omega 3 fatty acids for brain health.

Dr. Parker strongly encouraged changes in lifestyle—sleep, diet, exercise, motivation. He recommended that Mike get connected with a physical trainer and work toward three to four times a week of fairly vigorous exercise. He ended his recommendation with a sort of pep squad cheer: "Fight for brain health!"

As soon as the office door closed behind us, Mike said, "I'm not adding any more drugs to my body!"

"Well, you'd be taking one away, Topamax, and adding a stimulant."

"I don't have ADD! All he wanted to do was play cards!"

I encouraged Mike to follow up on Dr. Parker's suggestions for lifestyle changes. By this time, though, any encouragement from me only elicited resistance. Matt and Sharon both talked with Mike about getting more exercise and eating more sensibly. He always agreed that more exercise or a better diet would be a good idea, but that was as far as it went.

In October, after consulting with Dr. Bertoli and also with Dr. Carlson, Mike agreed to take Dr. Parker's advice, gradually drop Topamax, and, also gradually, add Ritalin to his daily drug intake. His mood and energy level were slightly improved with Ritalin, but not his difficulties in keeping track of things.

Clinging to the good news that whatever was up with Mike didn't follow an Alzheimer's pattern, I was also reassured by the results of his MRI. "Mild chronic sinus changes…. No evidence for acute sinusitis. Mild age-related changes of the brain. Otherwise, normal brain MRI."

In September, Mike entered a sleep clinic for an overnight polysomnography evaluation. The results showed mild sleep apnea. He was set up with a continuous positive airway pressure (CPAP) mask. A technician came to the house to walk Mike through the processes of using the mask and returned the following week to reinforce the practice. Although Mike assured the technician that all was going well and that he was sleeping with the mask on all night every night, he generally tried it for an hour or less, then set it aside.

Gradually, almost unconsciously, I'd been covering more and more details for Mike—helping him with email, keeping a backup calendar for his appointments, getting him to and from appointments, and generally watching out for whatever was next. He resented being "monitored," and I resented the time suck of monitoring, but Mike was losing too many details when left on his own.

Puttering around in the kitchen one afternoon, I heard the phone ring, then heard Mike telling the caller his Social Security number. I went to him and tapped him on the shoulder. "Who's that?" I mouthed. Mike glanced at me, then repeated the number. When he hung up I sat down beside him.

"It's not a good idea to give out your Social Security number on the phone," I said.

"It was just the bank."

"It could have been anyone," I said.

"It was the bank! Citibank! That's what she said!"

"The bank already has your Social Security number."

"They wanted to confirm!"

So now I needed to pay closer attention to phone calls, too.

In the category of paying closer attention, I was interacting with Mike's church choir singers in a way that I'd never done before—confirming rehearsal dates and times, calling Mike's attention to choir-related emails, even printing such emails out for him. I'd had hints from some of the choir members that rehearsals were sometimes disorganized. Nothing stated outright, but there was a subtext. One of the choir members, Susan Forester, was also on the staff as a part-time nurse. She and I had connected easily at choir parties, and I felt I could talk with her in confidence. I made an appointment and met with her in her office at the church. I told her I had some concerns that Mike was having difficulty keeping track of things, and asked if she had observed any such difficulties. She had.

She wondered if he might be having petit mal seizures. There were times when he would seem to blank out for an instant, then come back. He was less organized in rehearsal than he'd been the previous season. She emphasized how much they all loved Mike. What a wonderful musician he was, etc., etc. But yes, she and others were also concerned that something was wrong.

Notes from my very sporadic journal entries indicated the same behaviors at the end of December 2008, as those listed in 2007, though each of the behaviors had become more pronounced. What in 2007 had been "occasional indifference and self-absorption with others," was now constant rather than occasional.

Prescription drug intake had increased both in variety and dosage.

I had two of those plastic containers with divisions for each day of the week. One was clear, and on that I put a sticker-picture of the sun. The other one was dark blue, opaque, and I gave that a sticker-picture of the moon. But in spite of my efforts to help Mike know which pills to take in the morning, and which in the evening, he could no longer handle his meds on his own. In addition to keeping track of his calendar, helping him with email and all things computer related, seeing to it that his car got serviced, and aiding communications with him between both church choir and Chanteuses singers, I was now managing his meds—refilling prescriptions, putting pills in weekly plastic containers, doling them out first thing in the morning and before bedtime, and hiding the containers between times.

ANOTHER WRINKLE
IN TIME
2008

It is November. I'm returning home from San Antonio after the annual National Council of Teachers of English conference and the following Assembly on Adolescent Literature workshop, where I spoke on the subject of Intellectual Freedom in teen fiction. Since the conference included a weekend and Mike had choir duties, I went on my own.

My plane lands in Sacramento late Tuesday night, and I make my way down to baggage claim, where Mike usually meets me and helps carry things to the car. When he isn't there, I assume he's decided to pick me up at the curb rather than bother to park. I get my bag from the carousel and schlep that, along with my oversized purse and computer bag with presentation materials, out front where I watch every gold Honda come around the curve, hoping it is ours. After 20 minutes or so I call Mike's cell phone but as is often the case, it isn't turned on. I call our home phone. Mike answers, sleepily.

"Are you in bed?" I ask.

"Yes. I was tired."

"I'm waiting for you at the airport."

"I thought you were getting in tomorrow night."

"No, hon. I'm here now."

"Okay. I'll be right there."

"I'm at the curb, outside Southwest baggage claim doors."

It is indicative of my growing acceptance that Mike can't keep dates straight that I didn't bother to point out to him that my itinerary had been front and center on the refrigerator, with another printed copy on his desk, and also in his email file, and that I'd called him from the airport just that morning, before I left San Antonio. It was also indicative of my changed expectations that I'm not angry, just very, very sad.

Mike arrives about a half hour later and puts my bags in the trunk without a word. On the way home he complains of how tired he is. I try to give him a few highlights of the conference, but he can only turn the "conversation" back to being tired. Once home he deposits my suitcase in the utility room and goes upstairs, again without a word. A very different welcoming than those of just a few years ago, when, after carrying my bags upstairs, he would pour champagne, set out brie and crackers, maybe a few bunches of grapes, and we would talk long into the night of what had gone on with him in my absence, and of the details of my experiences away.

Although I seldom watched TV, I did that night, knowing I was too stirred up for sleep to come soon. Sunny curled up beside me on the couch, with her head resting on my thigh. I found an old Carol Burnett show and was soon laughing at the antics of Tim Conway. After an hour or so, Sunny and I went upstairs to bed. Within moments, Mike snuggled close against my back. "Love you big time," he muttered sleepily. It was sweet, but it didn't mean as much as it once had.

ALWAYS
2009

Saturday, March 7, 2009: Not quite awake, I lie close against Mike's back, matching the rhythm of my breathing to his. Hints of sunlight filter through tiny gaps in the shutters of our upstairs bedroom. He rolls over to face me. A sweet, sleepy kiss on my forehead and then, "I love you."

"I love you, too," I tell him, stroking his cheek.

Hovering just below the surface of fully awake, it's as if things are as they've always been. We love each other. We are partners in each other's lives, living out the "for better or worse" we both promised over four decades ago, with the scales mostly balanced on the side of "for better."

We kiss again, this time a lingering kiss on the lips, something that could, perhaps, lead to more, though between Mike's antidepression meds and my past-prime vagina, "more" is a place we don't often visit. Still, the slight stirring is welcome and prolongs the illusion that things are as they've always been.

As with most signs of troubles that come to other people at other times—the barely discernible lump near the left armpit, the empty bottles of cheap whiskey wrapped in newspaper and buried under other trash on pick-up day—Mike's recent cognitive gaffes allowed for an interpretation of benign causes, and I, not wanting to see what I was seeing, attributed missed appointments to his not caring enough to write things down. When we planned to meet for dinner at 6 o'clock at Chevys and he went to Casa Ramos instead, I was pissed that he hadn't bothered to get even that simplest of plans straight. Then came the Daylight Saving Time fiasco.

On this Saturday morning, before our clocks are to "spring ahead," Mike insists on setting his watch and every clock in the house forward an hour.

"Let's wait until just before bedtime," I say. "The time doesn't officially change until 2 tomorrow morning."

"I know," he says, proceeding to reset all of the clocks.

Throughout the course of the day Mike believes that he alone has the correct time. When I suggest otherwise, he points to the clock in the kitchen as proof that what I and the rest of the western states are thinking is 2 in the afternoon is really 3. Troubling as this is, it makes no difference in our practical world until a little after 5 in the evening. We've just been served margaritas and dinner at our local Mexican restaurant when, after a quick look at his watch, Mike announces that it is time to go.

"The show doesn't start until 7," I say, taking the "River City Cabaret" tickets from my purse and pointing to the listed time.

Mike looks at the tickets.

"Dessert and drinks at 6:30," he says.

"Okay, so we have an hour and a half, and the Elks Lodge theater is only 10 minutes away."

Mike taps his watch. "6:15" he says, and calls for the check.

The waiter hurries to our table.

"Is anything wrong with your order?"

"No," Mike says, reaching for his American Express card. "We have tickets to a show, and we don't want to be late."

When the waiter returns with our card, I ask him if he can give me the time.

He glances at the clock over the bar.

"5:15," he says.

When he's out of earshot I say to Mike, "See, it's really only 5:15. The time hasn't actually changed yet."

Mike gets up to leave.

"Please don't do this. Let's just enjoy our margaritas and have a relaxed dinner."

"I'll be in the car," he says, and walks out.

I take a few more sips of margarita, another bite of spinach enchilada, but it's no use. I leave the restaurant, get in the car, and ride in angry silence to the Elks Lodge.

The woman at the ticket desk tells us it will be an hour or so before the theater doors open, but we can wait in the dining room if we'd like.

We follow her directions to a large room filled with white-clothed tables that are apparently waiting for diners. There's a small bar set up in the corner, complete with a bartender. The capacity sign on the wall allows for 320, but at

5:30 there are only the three of us in the room.

"Would you like a glass of Merlot?" I ask Mike.

"No, thanks. I'll have something when we go inside."

I order a glass of Chardonnay and we sit at one of the tables. We comment on the room and the surprising largeness of the whole facility. We've driven past it hundreds of times but never really paid much attention.

After a few minutes of trivial conversation Mike decides to go back to the theater. Although it's still a long time before the doors are to open, I don't bother to say so.

"I'll be in after I finish my wine," I say.

From a rack near the bar, I gather printed information on Elks activities and take my collection back to the table. On the blank back page of an Elks brochure I write a frenzied account of my anger and frustration—Mike's stubbornness, my missed dinner, this wasted time, Mike's unwillingness to consider anyone else's point of view, etc., etc.

Finally, another glass of wine and three defaced brochures later, puzzlement overcomes anger. I think back to other events of the recent past—going to his church choir directing job on Saturday, thinking it was Sunday, then being angry that no one had shown up. Missing a dress rehearsal for a small choral concert in which he was the tenor soloist. Showing up for a doctor's appointment a day early. Calling the newspaper on a Tuesday morning to complain that the Sunday *New York Times* had not been delivered.

What I have not wanted to see flares before me like the blinding bright lights of an oncoming car on a dark country road, and I know in the depths of my being that Mike's sense of time has been ripped apart, as if it has gone through one of those cross-cut paper shredders, and there is nothing either he, or I, or anyone else can do to paste it together again. A sense of impending disaster fills my consciousness, casting all else aside. Our upcoming trip to Florida? The dry rot in our patio eaves? Tomorrow's manicure appointment? Our 3-year-old granddaughter's sudden emergence as a master of the English language? All such thoughts of the everyday joys and challenges of life are but grains of sand, buried deep beneath the avalanche of impending doom.

I sit at the table, surrounded by all of those other empty tables, practicing deep breathing, practicing the serenity prayer, practicing detachment. Finally, as a distraction, I read the front of the first sullied brochure, surprised to see that the Exalted Ruler of the lodge is a woman. I fantasize briefly about joining the Benevolent and Protective Order of Elks. They offer a number of significant scholarships each year. As a retired teacher I'm all for supporting education. We could come to the Wednesday night spaghetti dinner for only $5. I like the bartender.

After a brief time in the Elkland fantasy, I remind myself that I'm not the club type and go in search of Mike. The doors to the theater are now open, and people are gathering at tables and lining up for drinks and desserts. I find Mike at a table near the stage. "Here, I saved you a place," he says, smiling, as he stands to pull the chair out for me.

Halfway through the show, a small ensemble sings a song that, for all its overdone familiarity, still conjures cherished memories of our shared history. "… I'll be loving you, always, with a love that's true, always …" Mike reaches for my hand. With the warmth of his long-familiar touch, I rest my head lightly against his shoulder.

"… Days may not be fair, always. That's when I'll be there, always …"

Melody and memory fill me with the sweetness of so many times past—newly married, dancing in the lounge of the Century Plaza Hotel in Los Angeles. A few stolen moments with the old VM hi-fi, kids finally asleep. Mike's brief glance my way from the Pasadena coffeehouse stage, as he sang in his strong, pure, tenor voice "… Not for just a year, but always …"

On the way home, Mike suggests that, since we don't have to worry about getting up early in the morning, we stop for dessert.

"Didn't you say you called the choir for an early rehearsal tomorrow?"

"Not tomorrow," he says. "Tomorrow's Saturday."

"No. Tomorrow's Sunday."

"Saturday," he says, turning onto the street of his favorite pie and coffee place.

Mike orders a piece of apple pie with ice cream and a cup of decaf coffee, as he always does. I order a cup of real coffee with cream, as I always do. But, as I learned in my long ago English major days, "the moving finger writes; and having writ, moves on…" and the bold, indelible writing on this page of my life declares that "as always" is no longer, and will never again be.

June 2012

Dear Mike,

I hardly ever have occasion to use Sunrise anymore, that congested thoroughfare we once used on a daily basis, Gold River to the freeway, or up to Macy's or Trader Joe's. But yesterday I decided to browse Christopher & Banks for a new summer T-shirt. It's strange how very familiar yet foreign that part of the area now seems.

Waiting for the signal to change, a gold 2005 or so Honda Accord turned left from Gold Country Boulevard onto Sunrise. Sunroof open, man sitting tall behind the wheel. Your area. Your car. Your posture. In that millisecond of recognition my heart stopped, quickened, then fell. How is it that you can be absent for so long, then suddenly come to me in the guise of a stranger in a strange car? And how is it that I still expect you? Whenever will my unconscious feeling self catch up with the conscious thinking self that knows you are gone, that you are never coming back to that corner, that car, that posture?

Unlike the old days, I now have the cheapest cable service possible and so don't find much of interest on TV. But I allow myself the luxury of a basic Netflix membership. Last night I watched "The Iron Lady" on a Netflix DVD. I'd missed it when it came out in 2011. Having never been a fan of Margaret Thatcher's politics, I was mainly interested in seeing it for Meryl Streep's Academy Award-winning performance. The movie is framed by the older Margaret Thatcher in the early stages of dementia, with flashbacks to her earlier life and the high and low points of her reign as prime minister. It was a compelling production with any number of poignant scenes, but the scene that brought me to tears was when the older Thatcher was going through her long dead husband's closet, determined to finally get rid of his clothing. I started crying when she buried her face in his tuxedo.

How hard it was for me to send your tuxedo to the consignment shop. Your tuxedo, so indicative of you, still with a hint of your scent if I buried my face deeply enough into the jacket. So hard to part with.

My tears didn't last long. The scene soon shifted and with it my attention. Like life.

I still have your pitch pipe in the middle drawer of the desk that used to be yours, but that I now use. The desk from my old office was much too big for my present scaled-down life. Matt now has my old desk in his office in Walla Walla. But your pitch pipe, in its little red velvet pouch, still sits in the middle drawer. It takes up so little space and still, in a way, holds the spirit of your lips, your breath. Your clothes, though, are gone.

Tomorrow I'll bring cookies, and a picture of Lena and her band, and a picture of Subei at graduation. You will likely look at each one for just an instant, then put them on the hall table on your way out. Maybe you will pick them up again on your next round, then place them on one of the living room shelves as you complete a loop. I don't think the pictures will mean anything to you, but who knows? I'll give it a try. Just in case.

Still missing you,
Marilyn

CHRISTMAS IN LAGUNA

2008

A week or two before Christmas I asked Mike to take the Honda in for servicing, in preparation for our trip to Southern California.

"I'm not going," he said, but he took the car in.

The Saturday before we were to leave, I got out our suitcases from the garage and suggested to Mike that he pack a few things.

"I'm not going."

Sunday, while Mike was at church, in addition to my own bag, I packed a bag for him. I know a lot of wives regularly pack for their husbands, but this was a first for me. Long trip, short trip, it didn't matter. Mike always packed his own bag. He was particular about his clothes, and also about how they were folded in the suitcase. In the past, in preparation for some trip, I'd spread the clothes I wanted to take out on the bed, and Mike would pack for me, too. Not lately, though.

Early Monday morning, I carried our suitcases downstairs and began loading the car with gifts. Mike stood watching.

"Can you grab a few Christmas CDs?"

He disappeared into the house, then returned with a box of 10 or so of our favorites. We plucked a few treasured ornaments from the tree Mike had decorated more than a week ago, and grabbed garland and a string of lights from a box of unused Christmas things.

"I don't know why you're doing this," Mike said.

"Just for a change."

"I'm not going!" he said, standing stiff, fists clenched, head thrust forward as if preparing to fight.

"Matt and Leesa and Mika will be there."

"I don't know why you're doing this!" he said, still stiff and tight.

"Grab a few bottles of water for us, would you?"

He gave me a long look, then turned and went inside. He returned with four bottles of water and some potato chips.

"Thank you."

I put my arms around him and held him tight.

"I love you. This is going to be a good time," I told him.

"I don't think so," he said, but when I got into the driver's side of the car, he walked around to the passenger side and got in.

Several times on the way down Mike repeated his "I don't know why you're doing this" mantra. Each time I named each person who would be there. As was our practice on trips south, we stopped for lunch at Harris Ranch and switched drivers. I held my breath as we approached the freeway overpass, hoping against hope that he wouldn't take the northbound onramp in the direction of home. I breathed a huge sigh of relief as he passed the "North to Sacramento" ramp and took the entrance south toward Los Angeles.

We got to the Aliso Creek Inn mid-afternoon, unpacked and went shopping for a Christmas tree. The one we found was scrawny in comparison to our usual trees, but it was the right size for our small condominium living room. To the accompaniment of Mario Lanza singing "O Holy Night," Mike carefully unwrapped the Lladro Baby's First Christmas ornaments he'd bought for each grandchild. They were white porcelain, an infant in a stocking, with "Baby's First Christmas" and the year printed across the top of the stocking. Ashley, 1991. Kerry, 1993. Subei, 1995. Lena, 2001. Mika, 2006. He announced each one as he carefully placed it on the tree.

After decorating, we went to the Scandia Bakery and ordered a birthday cake for Dale—chocolate with a gooey strawberry filling, white icing decorated with red poinsettias and "Happy Birthday Dale" in big, red letters.

"I always do the dessert," Mike said.

"I know. But this will work, just this once."

The others began arriving the next day and the mood was festive. The Southern California warmth was a welcome change from the winter chill of our home territories. In the afternoon we all walked to the beach. There was a little park between the public parking lot and the beach, and Subei and Lena took Mika down the highest slide at the play structure. When they tired of that, the two older kids slid down sand dunes as if on snow sleds. Uncle Matt showed Subei a particularly impressive soccer move and threw his back out. It was reminiscent of the time Uncle Dale's back took a hit while accompanying young Matt down one of those giant slides at the fair, the kind you ride down on burlap bags. What great, self-sacrificing uncles we have in our family!

We found shells at the water's edge and talked of past times at Aliso Creek. This group, plus longtime friends of ours, had celebrated our 20th anniversary here on this beach. Dale, though, was sick in bed on that long ago night. After champagne and hot dogs around the fire pit, Mike and our friends, also singers, went back to the condo and serenaded Dale with rousing Baptist hymns, claiming there was healing power in the lyrics none of us any longer believed in, "Power in the Blood," etc. Maybe it worked. The next morning Dale was up and about, feeling fine.

We'd been at this same place in the summer of 1995, when Sharon and Doug got word that there was a baby waiting for them in China. There was basic faxed information, including a picture of a tiny baby girl with a mass of black hair combed into what looked like a mohawk. We'd gathered around the picture, Sharon, Doug, Dale, Marg, Corry, Mike and I, laughing and crying, already loving the baby whose name we didn't even yet know. Mike took off abruptly, then returned an hour later with a frilly red baby dress and matching booties.

Then there was the Fourth of July when Mike nearly got arrested for fireworks on the beach. And the time Doug saved me from drowning. Later, whenever he'd found me to be particularly annoying, he would wonder aloud why he'd been so quick to drag me from the water. We were amused and buoyed by layer upon layer of past times at Aliso Creek, even as our present experiences were tainted by changes in Mike.

Mike and Mika built a sand castle, and later watched "Singin' in the Rain" together. We all went to dinner at Las Brisas, another place that was laden with memory. The mood was light and festive, and Mike finally seemed to accept our shift in tradition.

Christmas Eve morning I drove Mike to John Wayne airport. In the pocket of his jacket was the printout for a rental car, return flight information, and lists of times when he needed to be at church.

"We won't open one single gift without you," I promised.

"When do I get back?"

"I'll pick you up here, outside Baggage Claim, at 1:30."

"Promise?"

"Of course, I promise."

I told him I loved him, that I hoped the concert would be wonderful, asked that he call once he got home, and kissed him goodbye.

All seemed to go smoothly. We talked that night around 10:30. Mike was pleased with the concert—said the choir had sung beautifully and that they sailed past the weak spots he'd been worried about.

Christmas morning, I managed to sit parked for a few minutes outside Baggage Claim and was waiting at the curb as Mike walked out. He was happy—eager to get back to the Christmas festivities. By 2:30 we were all gathered in the funkily decorated Aliso Creek living room, ready to open gifts.

Several years ago our Christmas drawing practices had shifted from buying gifts for whomever we'd drawn, to donating to a charity in that person's name. It was always interesting, sometimes inspiring, to learn what charities had been chosen as gifts. Heifer International, National Wildlife Federation, Sacramento's Loaves and Fishes, SPCA, Save the Children, etc., etc. We still gave tangible gifts to the grandkids, but they also participated in the charity drawing. It seemed to be more in keeping with the spirit of Christmas than the overblown indulgence earlier Christmases had morphed into.

In the evening we put candles on the decadent cake and shifted themes from Christmas to birthday. It was a full and happy day. Later that night, in bed, Mike allowed as how it had been a good Christmas, but he wanted next year to be back at our house.

"This was just a one time deal," I assured him.

I was nearly asleep when he said, "I never did find the headlight switch on that rented car."

So … 12 miles to the church at 7 p.m., already dark, to 12 miles home around 10 o'clock, no lights. Driving a rental car was another item that needed to be crossed off the list of things Mike could safely do.

May 23, 2012

Dear Mike,

Nancy Obrien died early this morning. I am so saddened by this news. Nancy, 62. Always so full of life, and energy, until just three months ago, when something in her body turned against her.

We should be wrapped in each other's arms, crying together on the martini couch, remembering some of our many times together, your growing friendship with her when the two of you were new to the Los Angeles Master Chorale. It probably wasn't until that walk through the Cotswolds back in 1990 that I, too, began to treasure her friendship. We should be crying together, and remembering, until our hearts lighten with laughter over some of those silly shared times. The little antique stores she would ferret out, to your delight and my dismay. And tea shoppes, with "biscuits" and clotted cream. Her way of finding a Catholic church to attend no matter where we were on a Sunday. We could be comforted by her practice now, knowing that she found solace in her faith to the very end. That's true. Jeanne D., who was with her all along, assured me of that.

It seems I can almost hear her singing "Danny Boy," as she sang it in that little B&B on the last night of our walk through the Ring of Kerry. Bill accompanied her on the dining room piano. That may have been the first time I truly appreciated Nancy's voice and musicianship. I'm afraid that whenever there was occasion for a little spontaneous music, I mostly only had ears for you. I know, "Danny Boy" is thought to be clichéd, especially by sophisticated musicians, but that night at Lough Leane was far beyond a cliché.

We should be saying these things to each other, Mike. There is no one else in this world with whom I have such a wealth of shared memories. I miss you so much right now.

Later today I will visit you at Porto Sicuro. I will see the picture of you and Bill and Nancy taken at her 60th birthday party at the Arcadia arboretum. That was the last trip you were able to make to Southern California on your own, and even then it took a lot of maneuvering at both ends to make it happen. I made all of the travel arrangements and saw you with ticket and ID in hand to the end of the security check line. Bill was waiting for you when you got off the plane in Burbank. The thought had been that you would rent a car while you were in town, but it became more and more apparent that you couldn't get that organized. Bill ended up taking you to see David, and the Sandboms, and generally watching out for you while you were there. You had already lost a big chunk of yourself by that time—I had lost a big chunk of you. Still, when I walk into your room and see that picture of the three of you smiling happily, I will long to have even that much back.

Marilyn

DIMINISHING
NEST EGG
2009

Winter and spring. Since the second year of our marriage we both realized we couldn't maintain a shared checking account. Mike was big on immediate gratification and would charge clothes and household items that I thought were beyond our means. I wanted to pay for everything when I bought it, not use credit. The result of our different approaches meant that on payday our money was already earmarked to pay Bullock's and Robinson's for Mike's previous month's purchases. Endless discussions, attempts at budgets couldn't solve these differences because "budget" was a concept lost to Mike, and our different approaches to money was a source of great frustration for us both. The only answer seemed to be separate checking accounts, and that mostly worked for a long time.

From my teaching income, and later book business income, came all basic household expenses, food, utility bills, my car expenses and, if I were in the process of buying a new car, those payments. From Mike's teaching income and music jobs he paid the house payment, his own car expenses, entertainment, his charge accounts. We combined resources for larger items of furniture, travel, Christmas gifts and parties at our home, etc. Mike paid the vet bills. I paid for the newspaper delivery. Over time I succumbed to the convenience of credit cards but paid them off every month.

It's an illusion to think there is such a thing as separate finances in a marriage, especially a marriage in a community property state like California, but it was an illusion we maintained for decades. Now, though, I found I needed to pay attention to Mike's part of the finances as well as my own—watching the mail for past due notices, trying to make sense of argumentative calls with his bank. In the past if we went to dinner with friends, Mike paid our half of the bill and tip. Now he often didn't bother to get cash for such an evening out, and if he paid with a credit card, he neglected to add a tip. This in itself wasn't a big deal as long as I was paying attention; it simply was another puzzling change.

In addition to a significant loss in value of our retirement funds with the recession, the equity in our Gold River house had dwindled to just barely above a break-even point. We'd also taken income hits. Mike's Northminster choir job paid less than his previous music director's job had. Because school budgets had been hit so hard with the downturn, there was no longer money for "enrichment," which was the category under which my books fell. Book royalties were suddenly down by 50 percent. Money for school visits and teacher workshops had also been drastically slashed. Where for the past six or seven years I'd had 15 or so well-paying events a year, 2008 brought less than half that many, and 2009 was looking even more bleak.

I quit getting regular manicures. I switched from the upscale Gold River hairstylists to Supercuts. Drugstore cosmetics. Occasional drive-through car washes rather than regular visits to the nearby custom car wash. House cleaners only rarely instead of every other week. Cheaper restaurants. Too little. Too late.

In 2009, shortly after the first of the year, I took over all of the banking and bill paying tasks. Mike barely noticed the change. I was disheartened to learn that we still owed more than $19,000 on Mike's car, the Honda Accord we'd bought five years earlier. We'd used an equity loan for the purchase, and, unbeknownst to me, Mike had only been paying the minimum, the interest, for the past five years. He'd also been paying only the minimum on every bill for which he'd been responsible—Macy's, the gas card, Citibank, MasterCard, etc.

Over the years, the only credit card I used was my American Express, paid off each month. This was a time when credit card companies were sending offer after offer for low interest cards with which a high card might be paid off. Offers I had typically tossed into the trash without opening, I now began accepting. Thus began the shuffle of borrowing from Peter to pay Paul. I knew it was a slippery slope, a stopgap measure. But short of taking money from our retirement savings, already worth much less than it had been a year ago, I didn't know what else to do.

We needed to make significant changes to cut our expenses and live within our means. I began talking with Mike about selling our house and getting into something smaller with lower taxes, lower maintenance, lower or no homeowner association fees—maybe we should even consider renting. Mike's response was always the same. "I'm going to die in this house!" After hearing that one too many times, I suggested that if he were serious about dying in this particular house, he'd better hurry up—just one of many times I fell short in the love and compassion category.

Mike had been seeing Dr. Bertoli on a weekly basis for a year or more. He seemed to connect with her, though, except for the time immediately following a session, there didn't appear to be any change in Mike's up and down levels of depression. On the few occasions that I'd joined Mike with Dr. Bertoli, I saw that he paid closer attention to what I was saying when we were in that office than he did anywhere else. I set up a time to see Dr. Bertoli with Mike. Maybe she could help me convince him that we needed to take drastic measures to get our finances in order.

Looking back from my present vantage point, spending $500 a month for Mike to see a cognitive therapist was ludicrous. A *cognitive* therapist? Talk about money down the drain. At the time, though, it presented hope for a possible fix for whatever was wrong, and I was desperate for a fix.

It was around the middle of February when we sat together in Dr. B's office, and I gave a shortened version of why we needed to sell the house. She listened carefully to my assessment of our finances, listened carefully to Mike's determination to live out the rest of his life in our present house. She asked the right questions. Mike was focused and apparently open to making substantial changes.

Dr. Bertoli reminded Mike that he loved a new project. Would at least part of making a move be challenging and exciting? He allowed as how it would. By the time we left Mike agreed to pursue other possibilities. But when, a few days later, I suggested we look at some smaller places he was back to, "I'm going to die in this house."

May 2016

Dear Mike,

It's 8:15, turning from dusk to dark. I'm sitting in my little patio, having finished a glass of wine and the handful or more of cashews I'd put into a small ceramic bowl, part of a set you'd brought back from Japan. Were there once four of these? I'm not sure. However many you brought home, two now sit in the cupboard you've never seen, in the duplex you've never seen. You often came home from your travels with things that were too ornate for my tastes. But I've always loved these small ceramic bowls. Just the right size for melted butter on artichoke night, or for sour cream on baked potato night. They're grey, with random flecks of brown, and two muted circles of red near the lip of the bowl—again of a seeming random design. It's all random, isn't it? But I'm determined not to babble on about randomness, at least not right now.

What I wanted to tell you about is this very sweet evening, in this very pleasant place, this place you've never been. I'm sitting on one of the set of four outdoor chairs that sat around the table on the deck in Altadena, and around the table on the front patio in Gold River, and around Joe and Kathy's table in Rescue during that time when I had no place for a table around which to place them. How sturdy they've been—still are! I appreciate sturdiness, showing up for work every day, uncomplainingly getting the job done. I don't remember where they came from—maybe that huge Japanese nursery in San Gabriel that also had patio furniture and garden decor? Or maybe it was Monrovia. The place of purchase is lost to me now. I'm sure we chose the chairs together, though. With very few exceptions, we always chose furniture together, even though the choosing was complicated by our divergent tastes.

Securely attached to cross supports of the fence that separates my place from the neighbor's to the north is that large, bas-relief plaque depicting two angels. I think it's an image from a Raphael painting, though I'm not sure. Sharon gave this to us one anniversary, maybe our 35th. For several years it hung on a wall in our back patio at Promontory Point. Because it was a sort of terra-cotta color, it was somewhat lost against the sort of beige color of the wall. Then we had Sol, our favorite, perfectionist painter, paint a large, deep-purple circle on the wall as background for the angels. Glancing at the plaque now, which is not framed by a purple circle but by a grape stake fence, I'm guessing the dimensions are about 2½ feet wide and 1½ feet high. So many things fell by the wayside during the extreme downsizing from Promontory Point, but I'm glad the angels are still with me.

There is the "Follow the Yellow Brick Road" sign, a quotation from one of your favorite Yip Harburg shows, and the rough, grey, ceramic, wrinkled faces from The Gifted Gardener, another anniversary gift from us, to us. We liked the crusty old couple, he winking at her in what we interpreted as a playful, slightly lecherous manner. The bird feeder stand, the wicker chairs, the gardenia, the rose bush in the giant blue-glazed ceramic pot, all are from our old lives together.

Although I know all of the warnings about drinking alone, and am aware of my genetic disposition toward alcohol addiction, in the evenings I continue to have a glass of wine, or two, as we used to do together. When I sit on this patio, with wine and cheese, or nuts, the surroundings and fare are reminiscent of times with you. But I am not maudlin. My thoughts as I sip and munch are of the day that has just passed, and the day that is to come. Maybe I think about my next task with a writing group I'm leading. Or the chapter I'm currently working on for this potential book. The kids, other family, friends, things as mundane as the need, soon, to give the bathroom a good scrub, or to pay bills … such are the thoughts that accompany my now solo version of cocktail hour. But as based in the present as such times are, they exist in the midst of representations of past times with you. As with the Raphael plaque or the wrinkled, winking faces, if I choose to bring these representations out of the background and into the foreground, the clarity of what we once had, and what we lost, emerges. That's a choice that I make sparingly.

But thank you again for so many of those times.

Marilyn

I THOUGHT
THEY LIKED ME

2009

In March, the minister of Northminster called to ask that Mike and I meet with him and Susan, the campus RN, to talk about choir-related issues. We did. They opened with a heartfelt prayer, an unintentional reminder to me that I was in foreign territory. But foreign territory or not, I knew they were sincere.

The minister and nurse both reassured Mike that they loved him and that they wanted to help make things work however they could. But too many issues had arisen that were getting in the way of the previously smoothly functioning choir.

The minister said that several choir members had come to him expressing their concerns about Mike. At times he seemed to lack focus. They also complained that he would repeatedly rehearse a number scheduled for months away and neglect pieces for the coming Sunday. Scheduling was a mess. He wasn't communicating with the Hand Bell director, which made her job more difficult. Was Mike aware of any of these difficulties?

Mike said he wasn't aware of any of that. He looked truly puzzled. Then he launched into a lengthy and detailed story of his baptism at the age of 11, the immersion, and the expectation that his life would change dramatically. He also talked about being raised Southern Baptist, no cards, no alcohol, etc., etc., etc. The minister tried to get back to the topic at hand. The nurse gave a few examples of times when things had gone awry. Did he remember when they had to rearrange his music for him? No, he didn't, and then it was back to his baptism.

The meeting lasted over an hour and when we got into our car to go home, Mike said, "I have no idea what that was about!"

I repeated a few of the concerns they had expressed in the meeting. Mike again said, "I have no idea what that was about."

At the time, I thought Mike was simply refusing to be interested in any point of view other than his own. Another example of his growing self-absorption.

What I suspect now is that he truly *didn't* have any idea what the meeting was about. He'd lost the capacity to understand any of the issues they'd raised.

The Chanteuses singers were also struggling to come to grips with how to deal with Mike's lessened musical competence. As with the church choir, I now often received emails confirming certain dates and times. At first this date-checking was occasional, then gradually they relied more and more on my back up for times, dates, and, ultimately, trying to keep Mike's music organized in his folder. I'd also begun meeting with one or two of the Chanteuses' leaders for coffee and, as with family, our talk centered on Mike's atypical behavior.

The preparation for their spring concert sounded as if it were grueling. One of the things the group had appreciated in Mike was that he challenged them to take on more complicated music and arrangements than they had done with previous directors. During one of our coffee conversations the two leaders agreed that Mike had taken them to a whole new level. But now he was having trouble with the rhythm of a particular piece. Someone had to keep track of his music for him, making sure it was organized in his folder. With the concert less than two weeks away, they'd given up hope that he'd get the rhythms right on that one piece. They decided to have him sit that number out. I don't remember what excuse they gave him, or who, if anyone, would be directing, but they felt they had no other choice.

This would be Mike's last concert with Chanteuses. The decision to let him go had been agonizing, and they had probably waited longer than they should have, but they loved Mike so much … they were so sorry about his lessening abilities … we sat in the bright cafe, the three of us giving way to tears. We puzzled over the possible causes of Mike's decline. I told them I'd asked for a referral to a neurologist, but the wheels were turning slowly.

On the day of the concert, Mike's skewed sense of time had him in his tux just a little after 9 in the morning.

"You don't need to be at the church until 5:30," I told him. "It's too early to be in your tux."

"Oh, okay," he said, going downstairs.

I followed behind, watching him pick up his music folder and car keys.

"It's not time yet, hon. Why don't you change clothes, and I'll take you out to breakfast?"

"I don't know what's happening," he said.

"Well, the concert starts at 7. You've asked the singers to meet you at the church at 5:30. That's eight hours away. We've got plenty of time for breakfast out, time to run errands, you know, the usual."

"I don't know what's happening!"

"I just told you!" I said, knowing as soon as my impatient words were out that to tell Mike first we do this, then we do that, was ridiculous because apparently he could no longer understand time sequences. I knew that, but in my impatience I forgot. I gentled my tone.

"Let's go upstairs. I need to change clothes, too."

He slammed his music and keys down on the counter and rushed upstairs where he stripped off his jacket and flung it on the bed, same with his pants and shirt.

I got out of my sweats and into something just a slight step up, hoping that Mike, too, would get into something more casual. He did.

"Come on, I'll take you to breakfast."

"I don't know what's happening!"

"Let's talk about it at breakfast."

The three-minute drive to Amore Cafe was tense and silent, but as soon as Mike opened the door to the restaurant he was all smiles. The owner greeted us as always, "How are you, my friends?"

"Great!" Mike said, full of enthusiasm. "How are you this morning?"

"Busy, but that's good."

"Good for you," Mike said, exuding warmth.

Could we just stay there until time for the concert? Keep Mike's public persona on the job?

I made breakfast last as long as possible, then did the same with errands. I took the long way to the bank, and to the cleaners. I stopped for gas, then ran the car through the car wash. There was a limit, though, to how long I could drag things out. It was just slightly after noon when we got home. Mike went upstairs and put on his tuxedo.

After many false starts—tuxedo on, tuxedo off, "I don't know what's happening," "It's not time yet," etc., etc.—I finally gave up sometime around 4:30.

I watched as he picked up music and keys for what seemed the thousandth time.

"Are you coming?" he asked.

"I'll be there before 7. I hope it goes well."

He turned, gave me a quick kiss, and was out the door.

Twenty or so minutes later he called from his cell phone.

"Well, I'm at the church, but nobody's here!"

"They're not due for at least another 15 minutes."

"Nobody's here!"

"Can you wait just a little longer?"

"They're not here!"

"Well … wait for me. I'll get there as soon as I can."

No matter what meds Mike was on, nothing seemed to alleviate his anxiety. As difficult as that was for me, it must have been infinitely more difficult for him.

Two of the singers were already there when I arrived, and they and Mike had started setting things up. I grabbed the book I was currently reading from the car and found a quiet place to sit in the church patio, but even the beautifully written, highly suspenseful *Story of Edgar Sawtelle*, could not win the battle for my attention when pitted against my growing fear of impending mishaps. As futile as I knew it was to dwell on worries, my attention was constantly drawn away from *Edgar Sawtelle* and back to Mike and to the Chanteuses group, and what likely lay ahead.

Over the decades I'd sat among countless audiences and congregations, watching the range of movements Mike used to communicate with singers. Whether a beginning or advanced high school choir, a raggedy or well-polished church choir or a group of professional musicians, Mike's conducting techniques didn't vary. His teaching techniques may have varied but not his conducting techniques. From head to toe, his whole body became an expression of the music before him. On the rare occasions when I'd been seated behind a choir and facing Mike, I'd marveled at his capacity to communicate with his singers through both broad and subtle gestures, facial expressions and eye contact.

For the sake of those around me, I've never sung in a choir. From the perspective of either a singer or choral conductor, I had little awareness of the finer points of delivering "Home on the Range," much less the Mozart Requiem. But I did know when I was witnessing a oneness of musical passion and purpose that reached beyond notes on a score or the technical expertise of singers.

From the early adoration of high school choristers to the ongoing respect of experienced singers, Mike was well thought of as a choral conductor. Several professional singers along the way told me of his precision as a director, his ability to deal fully with the depth and complexity of demanding works. Recently a man who had all of his life sung in choirs told me that Mike was the best director he'd ever experienced. "He made us better than we were," he said.

It's not likely that singers and fellow musicians would say to me, "Your husband sucks as a conductor," but the accolades rang true and expressed a reality that I could only intuit.

On that April evening at Trinity Cathedral, instead of finding a seat somewhere in the anonymous middle of the church as was my practice, I took a place in the pew directly behind where Mike sat waiting for the singers to enter. Why? Did I think I could suddenly jump up and right things in the likely event that something went wrong?

Usually the women of Chanteuses made their entrance projecting warmth, good cheer, and confidence. This evening their smiles seemed forced. There was a worried tension in the air. Maybe I only noticed this because I was so aware of troubles behind the scenes, but to me the tension was palpable. The singers were nervous. I was nervous. Mike, on the other hand, appeared to be more relaxed than he had been all day.

The opening number sounded a bit rocky, though again my expectations may have skewed my perceptions. Mike seemed unsure of the next number, shuffling through his music folder. One of the women in the front row stepped forward to find the piece for him. She made light of it and they went on. The next number Mike directed with the wrong piece of music in front of him, then sat down in the front pew.

"Not yet," one of the singers said, motioning him back. "You don't get to sit down until 'African Celebration.' After intermission."

"Oh. So am I directing this one?" Mike asked, standing to take his place. Again someone checked his music, found the next number and placed it in front of him. All of this was done with an appearance of lightheartedness, but I suspected I was not the only one there with butterflies in my stomach and sweaty palms. Several more times during this first half of the concert Mike sat down too soon, and the whole routine was repeated.

To my untrained ear there were very few places where things were obviously off. On one number Mike brought the singers in too soon, before the piano introduction was complete, and at other places I saw that the group was in charge, working around the uncertainty of Mike's leadership.

It was not until "Had I the Heaven's Embroidered Cloth," a Yeats poem set to music, that Mike truly rose to the occasion. I was again captivated by the fluidity of his body, the elegance of his gestures. And I knew for certain that this was the very last time I would ever see Mike conducting singers with such grace and precision, the nuances of his movements expressing the nuances of the music at hand. My throat tightened and I fought back tears, trying to hang onto the familiar scene that was, right then, passing from my life for all time.

Seconds after the last note of the Yeats piece, there was that faintly audible release of breath that comes with an audience's awareness that they have experienced the full power and mystery, the ultimate beauty of a unique composition, flawlessly performed.

Mike sat down.

Too soon.

After the April concert, the same two group members that I'd been meeting with met Mike for lunch. In a later conversation, they told me about their time with him. They'd spoken of their appreciation for all that he had done for them. They remembered good times. Then, in the gentlest way possible, they mentioned Mike's recent and puzzling difficulties keeping track of music, or dealing with complicated rhythms, or leading an organized rehearsal. They said they were shifting things around. In the fall they would be using another conductor.

When Mike returned home after that lunch, he'd stood at my office door. "They let me go," he said, his tone implying disbelief.

"Tell me about it."

"I guess they found someone they liked better."

"Is that what they said?"

"They let me go," Mike repeated, then went upstairs to bed.

Later, when he told others that he was no longer leading Chanteuses, he always said, "They like someone else better."

The following month, a few weeks after the church choir had sung their last service of the season, the minister called and asked if he and the nurse might meet with the two of us in our home.

"They want us to join the church," Mike predicted. "I'm not going to join the church."

I knew they were coming to ask that Mike take a "medical leave." I told him I thought it had to do more with things we'd talked about at our earlier meeting, things related to choir.

"I'm not joining the church," he said.

The minister and nurse arrived at 1 in the afternoon. We offered coffee, or tea, and cookies. We sat in the living room, Mike and I on the martini couch, the nurse and the minister each sat in one of the burnt orange barrel chairs. Then started the chit-chat. How lovely our house was, so nicely decorated, how long had we lived there, did we like it, how cute Sunny was, how old was she. I wanted to scream, "Just get the fuck on with it!" Instead I sat with my legs crossed, returning chit-chat with a frozen smile, while Mike threw in details of his baptism.

Finally, after much hemming and hawing, the minister said the choir had met and they all felt it would be best if Mike took a medical leave. They would love to have him back if and when his medical issues were resolved and he regained the competence needed to continue as choral conductor. They prayed with us. The nurse gave Mike a prayer shawl she had knitted for him, and they left. They'd been there for two hours that had seemed like two years. They were both very kind and sincere people, strong in their faith, and I could hardly wait to say goodbye.

Mike's puzzled response was, "I thought they liked me."

January 2011

Dear Mike,

I'm sorry. I wish I'd known early on that FTD was to blame for your lessened love—that it wasn't your fault. But by early 2006, your times of distance were coming more often and lasting longer. It was hurtful and maddening when you would walk out of the room while I was talking to you, or when you no longer bothered to greet me when we met at the end of the day. One scene still lingers.

The four of us, you, Jeannie, Bill and I, were meeting for dinner at 6 at Il Forno Classico. You had been at a choir related meeting at UUSS, and I had been sequestered in my office at home, working on yet one more draft of No More Sad Goodbyes. *You were already seated when I arrived. You stepped out so I could slide into the booth beside you.*

"How's your afternoon gone?" I asked.

"Same old thing," you said.

Your face had that tight, grey, sad look about it that let me know you weren't interested in conversation. I tried anyway. I mentioned a phone call with Sharon and talk of a possible visit from them. I told you I thought I was over the hump with Chapter Seven. When you didn't respond, I turned my attention to the menu.

We sat in silence until Jeannie and Bill came through the door. You stood to greet them, giving each a quick hug, your face bright and warm.

I don't remember the conversation. What I do remember is how animated you'd become with them, and how disengaged you'd been with me. Later, at home, I'd told you I wanted some of what you gave others.

"What do you mean?" you asked.

"I want some two-way conversation. I want your warmth and good cheer."

"You're my wife. I don't have to pretend with you," you said.

"Really?" I asked, but you were already out of the room.

I nursed my hurt, already losing the sense of your love that had so long sustained me.

Now, hanging on the wall to the left of my desk in the room you've never seen, is the colorfully stylized ceramic plaque you gave me years ago. "Save the Last Dance for Me," it says. Over the desk, high on the wall, is the sign you gave me one Valentine's Day: "Well-Behaved Women Rarely Make History." To my right is the framed art nouveau-style poster touting a production of Noel Coward's "Hay Fever." Noel Coward.

No one does Coward's "Mad Dogs & Englishmen" as well as you did—perfect comic timing. Reminders of you are scattered about. I don't know if that makes things easier or harder. Either way I'm missing you, missing us.

My love to you,
Marilyn

DIAGNOSIS
2009

In early June 2009, Mike and I met with Dr. Lee, a highly respected UC Davis neurologist. I had requested that Mike's medical records be forwarded, including the brain MRI and the neuropsychologist's report. As had become his pattern, Mike balked at "one more wild goose chase," but, with me chauffeuring, went when the time came.

Dr. Lee was thorough and honest, with a gentle manner. He put the MRI up on a screen and said he disagreed with the earlier interpretation of those results. There was significantly more damage than could be accounted for by "mild, age-related changes." He pointed to an area that showed signs of atrophy. I'm sure his explanation was clear and easily understandable, but I remember very little that he said beyond "significantly more damage."

Dr. Lee watched closely as Mike walked from one end of the room to the other. He did the usual physical exam—ears, eyes, nose, heart, lungs, reflexes. Then he proceeded with a series of questions and tasks, some of which our regular doctor had done with Mike, the usual count backwards by sevens, name the president, state the date, and some that were new.

Dr. Lee handed Mike an article from *Good Housekeeping* that told the story of two women, Emma and Martha, who had been close childhood friends in London, but had been sent to different regions of the English countryside during the blitz and had never reconnected. Then, more than 50 years later, there was a back page story in "The Guardian," complete with a picture, about Emma who, through a string of coincidences, had found a long lost locket that had belonged to her old friend. With the help of the Internet, she managed to get in touch with Martha. Though neither of them lived in London, they met at a hotel in that city and spent the weekend renewing their friendship. There were details about their families, careers, trials and successes.

Mike's confusion with dates and times was no surprise to me, but I was surprised by his response to the article. He read it through, out loud, perfectly.

Then Dr. Lee asked Mike to tell him about what he'd just read. Mike said it was about a locket that had been lost for a long time and then it was found.

"What were the women's names?"

"They found the locket."

"Where did they meet when they got together again?"

"It was an emerald."

"Do you know where the women lived as children?"

"It was on a gold chain." And so on.

Dr. Lee said he couldn't be sure what was going on with Mike. He doubted it was Alzheimer's. His guess was that it was some form of frontotemporal dementia. That was the first I'd ever heard the term. I wrote it down so I'd be sure to remember it. Dr. Lee recommended a brain PET scan, saying that because it measures brain activity, it would provide different information than the static picture of the MRI. Although it wouldn't offer a positive diagnosis of frontotemporal dementia, it would enable him to rule out Alzheimer's. Mike said he didn't want any more tests. There was nothing wrong with his brain. Dr. Lee very gently told Mike that something was going on that made it difficult for him to process information. He advised that we do everything possible to figure out what the source of his difficulties was, so that treatment might be possible.

"No more tests," Mike said. "There's nothing wrong with my brain!"

When they talked by phone later, Matt urged Mike to go for the scan, telling him something was wrong and it would be good to know what that was. If there were treatment, best to get that started right away. Mike finally agreed. I called Dr. Lee's office and asked that they order the scan.

Matt timed his July visit from Walla Walla so that he could go with us to our post-PET scan consultation with Dr. Lee. The three of us sat in a small, windowless examining room, facing the illuminated PET scan film clipped to a backlit screen. Dr. Lee said his first impression had been verified. There was no evidence of Alzheimer's. Everything pointed to early to mid-stage frontotemporal dementia (FTD). He explained that FTD affects the part of the brain that controls executive functioning—processes that have to do with self-management, self-control, planning, reasoning, judgment, inhibition, and more. My reasoning brain was thinking that explained a lot. My feeling self was rolling up into a tiny protective ball.

Dr. Lee informed us that the condition would get steadily worse, though it was impossible to say at what rate. There was no known treatment, but Aricept, a drug often used with Alzheimer's patients, sometimes appeared to slow the progression of FTD. Dr. Lee recommended that Mike get started with that.

"I'm not putting another drug into my system!" Mike shouted. "There's nothing wrong with my brain!"

With that he rushed out the door and down the hall. Matt and I made hasty goodbyes and rushed after him. In the car on the way home, Matt was able to reassure Mike, saying we would do everything we could to help deal with all of this. He encouraged Mike to at least try Aricept. As with the brain PET scan, it was Matt's influence that enabled us to get him started on Aricept.

Horrifying as the FTD diagnosis was, it also helped me, and others around us, to understand what was going on with Mike. Although I continued to be frustrated by Mike's distance from me, his repetitions, misinterpretations of events, inability to follow through with any decisions we made together, and his extreme inaccuracy in telling others stories of our lives together, I now knew that none of this was Mike's fault. In fact, "It's not his fault. It's not his fault" became an oft-repeated mantra of sorts.

When my patience was stretched thin by constant repetition, or by finding dirty dishes back in the cupboards before the dishwasher had been run, I would silently remind myself, "It's not his fault. It's not his fault. It's not his fault, no, it's not."

A variation of that chant was, "He can't help it. He can't help it. He can't help it, no, he can't."

Both of those phrases I chanted to the tune of Beethoven's "Ode to Joy," the same tune to which, back in 1967, I'd been escorted down the aisle by Dale, to take my place next to Mike.

As simplistic as the chanting routine sounds, it helped me kick up empathy and tamp down anger. Something that was sorely needed. The serenity prayer, yoga breaths, maintaining low expectations and watchfulness also helped me find patience. Not that I always found *enough* patience, but more than I would have had I not been working at it.

Having never even heard of frontotemporal dementia previous to our visits with Dr. Lee, I, along with close friends and family, began searching out and sharing whatever information we could find on that form of dementia. None of what we learned offered hope for Mike's future, or for my future with him.

In Doug's search for answers he found *What If It's Not Alzheimer's* and sent copies to me, Dale and Marg, and Matt and Leesa.

We read that people with FTD are sometimes "obsessed with a particular subject or event and that they will keep bringing the conversation back to this topic. Reminding the patient that they've already told the story many times before has no effect."

We were already witnessing such behaviors in Mike.

I searched the Internet for more clues about the nature of FTD, wondering what Mike might possibly be experiencing, trying to garner any hints as to what the trajectory of the disease might be. Wikipedia, the Mayo Clinic, the University of California, San Francisco, Memory and Aging Center—all said the same thing. There would be gradual and steady changes in behavior, increased language dysfunction, and/or, problems with movement. The rate of decline was unpredictable.

The websites that ultimately garnered most of my attention were the Association for Frontotemporal Degeneration and the FTD Support Forum. In the months that followed Mike's diagnosis, I checked the FTD Support Forum nearly every day, hungry to learn of how others were dealing with FTD, what symptoms they were observing in the person they cared for, how fast was the decline they were witnessing, what tactics were effective in dealing with difficult behaviors, etc., etc. Of course, no matter how often I checked the website, it didn't tell me what I most wanted to know. What course would the disease follow? What would be the time trajectory? But even though answers to my most pressing questions were not to be had, the personal stories gave me an awareness of how others were coping and helped me feel less alone.

A month or so after our visit to Dr. Lee, I sent a group email to friends and out-of-town family who had been expressing concern for Mike, telling them of the FTD diagnosis, that there was no cure or effective treatment, and that so far we were managing. People were amazingly generous with their expressions of concern and offers of help.

Sharon and Doug talked with friends and colleagues in health professions, the orthopedic doctor who shared space in their chiropractic office, a psychologist who was a close friend of Doug's, other doctors, nurses, caregivers. Marg used all of her nurse contacts to eke out any insights and information they might have. Dale talked with a good friend who had been caring for his parents for years and who had recently moved them into an assisted living facility. Cindi offered to move back to Sacramento from Nevada in order to help. Matt and Leesa stayed in close touch through email and phone calls, and, along with the others, asked the hard questions.

Sharon, Doug, Matt, Leesa, Dale and Marg all talked with me about the importance of being proactive. There would come a time when I was no longer able to take care of Mike. What then?

May 2013

Dear Mike,

Yesterday, Dale took me to the airport where I boarded a plane for Seattle, the first leg of the trip to Walla Walla. In Seattle, on the way to gate C2G, I was suddenly flooded with memories of our last trip together to Walla Walla. It was 2009, and although you had recently been diagnosed with FTD, you still were able to manage the basics—at least it seemed that way. But on that trip you abruptly left the table where we were eating lunch, saying you were going to the restroom. I sat at the table. Waiting. My mood shifting from mildly irritated to extremely worried. I tried your cell phone and got voice mail. I went to the gate where we were scheduled to depart for Walla Walla in about 45 minutes, thinking—hoping—you might have gone there without me. You weren't there. I spoke with an agent, who advised that I call the police, which I did. You don't need all of these details. Ultimately what happened was that the police located you and brought you to the gate where I was waiting. When you saw me you, called out, "I've been looking all over for you!" We were last on the plane, but we made it. In Walla Walla you disappeared from the bookstore, and the three of us, Matt, Leesa and I, searched the whole town for you. Eventually, I went back to the house while they continued looking. You'd been missing for nearly two hours when you came waltzing through the front door. "Where've you been???" you demanded.

I'm sorry. This is not what I want my focus to be. It's just that sometimes memories of such difficult situations overcome me.

This trip was uneventful. I walked through the doors of the Walla Walla airport and there was 8-year-old Mika, right in front, a huge smile on her face.

"Gramma!" she said, throwing her arms around me, giving me a long, tight hug.

On the way to the car, Leesa told me that Mika wanted to be my host and my servant during my stay.

"Only host," Mika said.

Back at their place Mika made a potholder from a kit I'd brought with me. She chose the colors and was careful to repeat a certain pattern. She told me she'd made one of those before. It wasn't her favorite thing to do, but she would do it for me. After dinner Mika gave a piano concert. She's doing well with the piano, and her current teacher's methods seem to work well with her. It's not the standard method of teaching notes and scales, but it gets kids playing songs from the very beginning, and I think that's particularly important for Mika.

It's beautiful here in Walla Walla, sunny and mild, with a light breeze. I walked into town this morning, admiring the array of color in so many well-tended yards. There's a place in front of my Sacramento duplex where Lloyd, my landlord, is going to tear out some ugly bushes to make room for new plants, so I'm getting ideas for what might best go there. It's mostly shady, so maybe azaleas or camellias, though I might like something a little less common. You would likely go for azaleas. What fun that was, when we first moved to Promontory Point and hired Kathy, the decorator-turned-landscape designer, to help with our patios. The professionally installed water fountain, the custom-made redwood trellis on which an espalier lemon tree would climb, artful stonework walkways, a densely planted carpet of wonderfully aromatic Corsican mint, a wall of jasmine along the side fence—$8,000 worth of patio upgrades. I could use that $8,000 now, but I wouldn't really trade it for the fun we had putting those patios together, and enjoying them on long summer evenings.

We weren't quite so extravagant when we moved two years later, two doors down, to the larger house. There was already a little pond in the front patio. You bought a beautiful pot, had a hole cut through the bottom, and added a pump that circulated water. The pond to fountain evolution was a long stretch beyond your natural talents and was a great success. Anyway, my mind is on a much lesser project of a new plant or two to brighten the front of my rented duplex.

I'm sorry that you can't be the quintessential grampa for Mika that you were for the other young grandkids. She is so like you in many ways. She's musical and loves to dance. She has a flair for fashion and drama. She knows, and expresses, exactly how she wants things to be. I know grandparents always think this, but I know it's true in her case—she's extremely intelligent. She and I love each other and have fun together, but you'd be doing tap dance routines with her, and playing dress up, feeding her way too many sweets, and doing your own quirky brand of improv with whatever stories you were reading and telling. How I wish you could be enjoying this amazing little person. How I wish she could have known you.

We miss you.
Marilyn

RETIREMENT COMMUNITIES

Fall 2009

With coaxing from those closest to me, I forced myself to get beyond the details of everyday life and consider both the immediate future, and what would likely need to be considered for the long haul. It was becoming more and more difficult to manage Mike. It was obvious I would soon need some sort of help.

On the advice of a social worker friend, Sharon contacted Carol Kinsel of Senior Care Solutions, a Sacramento organization that specializes in matching seniors with appropriate retirement facilities and also provides other resources for those necessarily difficult transitions. Sharon and I went together for our first appointment with Carol. She listened attentively, asked all the right questions, and helped us begin the process of navigating the stormy seas of caregiving for a loved one with dementia, coupled with growing financial instability. She provided us with an extensive list of local facilities, complete with information on costs and services, and also pointed us in the direction of another local organization, the Del Oro Caregiver Resource Center.

As with all other human services during this time of recession, Del Oro's budget had been slashed. At that time their resources to provide practical support to caregivers such as respite care, and free legal/financial consultations were severely limited. But their clinical consultant was able to secure, at a significant discount, the services of an elder attorney, to recommend a local support group that dealt specifically with issues of FTD, and to offer continued emotional and practical support through regular phone calls and emails.

Sharon, Dale, Marg, and I met with the elder attorney, Constance Hawkings. Matt participated with a conference call. Over the course of 90 minutes, Connie educated us about negotiating Medicare/Medi-Cal services, protecting assets, and getting remaining IRA accounts transferred to my sole ownership. We hashed over details of dealing with foreclosure, the advantages of bankruptcy—so many aspects of the legal system I'd never expected to need to know. I wish

I could somehow rewind the tape on that meeting and relive the specifics. My memory is that the whole thing was funnier than an SNL skit, though that seems rather far-fetched given the foreshadowing of disaster beyond disaster. I don't think our laughter was of the desperately hysterical type, but rather that we were all at the top of our form with irony and wit. Whatever the reality of the situation had been, thank the Goddess for convivial laughter.

By March, foreclosure notices started showing up in the mailbox. Where I had once blithely answered the phone whenever it rang, I no longer answered unless I knew for certain who would be on the other end when I picked up. I dreaded the mail. I dreaded the phone.

Armed with information from Senior Care Solutions, I began visiting local retirement communities. Maybe if we were somewhere that offered a lot of supervised activities, Mike would be easier to manage. I looked only at places that were three-tiered, offering independent living, assisted living, and memory care sections, thinking that Mike and I would be together in an independent living level apartment until it became necessary for him to move into a secure memory care section. When that time came, he would at least be familiar with that particular retirement community. When I found a place that seemed like a possible match, I did a second visit accompanied by Sharon and/or Dale and/or Marg, in whatever combination we could come up with. This was a huge decision, and the more observations and insights involved in the process, the better.

Even knowing it would be out of reach, Sharon and I first toured the Biltmore Plaza. This was not one of the facilities on Senior Care Solution's list of suggested places to visit. Their list was more realistically matched to my financial constraints.

We pulled into the circular drive, handed the keys to the valet parking attendant, and entered the living room/lobby that ran a close second to that of the San Francisco Fairmont hotel. We were met by Barbara, the marketing director, who led us to her spacious office where she asked about our specific needs in a senior assisted living community, gave us a basic overview of the Biltmore's offerings, then began the tour. She drew our attention to the living room's large fireplace, the comfortable conversation groupings, the card and game tables, the Steinway grand piano, and the aquarium. Other than the Monterey Bay Aquarium, this was by far the largest aquarium I'd ever seen. It was about 10 feet wide on both sides of the entry between the living room and dining room, and composed the upper half of the walls on each side. The two sides were connected by a wide, graceful archway, so that when we walked from the living room to the dining, room we could look up and see neon-colored exotic fish swimming overhead.

The Biltmore was proud of their "nationally renowned" chef and their "restaurant-style" anytime dining. We were invited to come back for lunch or dinner whenever we wanted, just call a day ahead of time.

The tablecloths were crisp white linen, the dinnerware again equal to that found in any luxury hotel. A variety of California wines were available if guests so chose. There was a lounge area with a full bar, complete with bartender. The bar was open daily for happy hour from 4 to 7 p.m.

"Most of our residents like to have their dinner any time from 4 to 5:30, though, of course, the dining room is open until much later for the few who prefer a later evening meal."

We met Lucy, the charming activities director, who told us of the huge variety of opportunities for recreation, pursuing special interests and hobbies. Every Sunday afternoon, live music was provided by members of one or another of Sacramento's many professional groups. Last week was the Chamber Orchestra; coming up was a group from the opera company.

The model apartment was beautiful but tiny.

"We like to encourage people to be out and about," Barbara said.

There was a gym and a brain fitness group, a quartet, writing groups, reading groups. If there wasn't a group we wanted, Lucy assured us she could help us start one.

The residents seemed happy and friendly. As we were leaving the model apartment, a woman chugging down the hall who looked to be somewhere in her 80s stopped to say, "Move in here! It's the best thing I ever did. More fun than a barrel of monkeys." She laughed, then moved on.

Back downstairs, there was a group playing bridge by the fireplace and another seemingly highly amused group playing something with dominoes, maybe Mexican Train.

After a tour of the large garden courtyard, comfortable seating areas and walking paths, we talked for a while longer in Barbara's office. We confessed that $9,000 a month was beyond our reach.

"Is your husband a veteran?" she asked.

"No."

"Long-term care insurance?"

"No."

She gave us the card of their social worker.

"Sometimes she finds ways of financing residencies that others have overlooked."

We left our contact information and said our goodbyes. As we drove away, Sharon said, "If Dad would like any of those places, he'd like this one."

I agreed. He would love the style of the place. "But can you picture us in that tiny apartment?"

Sharon laughed. "Yes, and it's not a pretty picture."

Next I visited Riverside. As at the Biltmore, the Riverside aquarium served as a divider between the living room and dining room, forming the upper half of the dividing wall to the right of the hallway, but not forming an archway or stretching across to the other side.

As the name implied, this place was close to the river. The grounds were fenced off, providing a secure parking lot with a gated entrance and exit. There was a pedestrian gate at the back of the property that allowed access to the river. I loved having easy access to the American River Parkway by way of the Gold River nature paths. It would be nice not to have to give that up.

As with the Biltmore, Riverside had restaurant-style dining and a well-credentialed chef. They had a full bar but, unlike at the Biltmore, their bartender was only on duty from 4:30 to 7 p.m. for Friday, Saturday and Sunday happy hours.

The marketing director was so charming, I thought we might become new best friends. I later realized that all marketing directors are charming, and there is always the implication that they might become one's new best friend, but this was only my second visit to a retirement "facility."

Riverside was considerably less per month than the Biltmore Plaza, but it still had an air of genteel refinement. In addition to liking the ambience, I was particularly interested in their brain fitness program. The exercises made use of previous common experiences with movies and music of our times, some political trivia, sports trivia, and other aspects of our common culture. I could picture Mike enjoying this program, and mightn't it keep parts of his brain active at least for a while? He had been a whiz at Trivial Pursuit. I always wanted him on my side for music and movies, history and politics, but he even often managed to come up with the answers to questions in the sports category—a surprise, since his main connection to sports was his annual viewing of Super Bowl halftime extravaganzas. Halftime only. He'd already be back to an old movie on Turner Classics before the kickoff for the second half of the game.

Sharon and I visited Riverside together, as did Dale and Marg and I. We all liked the look and feel of the place. Residents were friendly and cheerful. There was a grand piano in the lobby/living room and a small upright in the second floor gathering space. The perky activities director assured us that both pianos were tuned monthly.

Riverside would be around $5,000 a month. Considerably less than the Biltmore, but still hardly affordable. The truth, though, was that nothing would be affordable. Wherever we ended up, I would be dipping into what was left of our nest egg to meet monthly expenses—not a good long-term plan.

With the major exception of affordability, Riverside more than met our criteria. As with the Biltmore, the apartments were tiny. But there was a unit on the ground floor that had a little patio and an outdoor entrance. That was bound to feel less closed in. Friends could come to our front door from the parking lot. Sunny could still have a bit of outdoor space. It would feel less institutional to enter from the outside rather than walking through the living room, down the hall to the elevators, then up to the second or third floor and down another hall to our apartment.

It was all so uncertain. If Mike only had two more years on this earth, our IRAs would cover a nice place like Riverside—a place with a look and style that Mike might warm to—a place with activities that might be a good fit with his personality. I wanted Mike to be as happy and content as possible during his continuing deterioration. On the other hand, much more than two years at a place like Riverside would have us destitute.

I was sleepless with worry. Weighing and measuring alternatives was important and, ultimately, I hoped, productive. Endless worry was not. I made a conscious choice to tuck my worries into a compartment and only let them out once or twice a day. Of course, the lock on the compartment didn't always hold, but the practice helped me balance the tightrope between necessary action and despair.

THE DOWNHILL SLIDE BECOMES AN AVALANCHE

July through December 2009

Our financial situation was becoming increasingly difficult. It was a stretch to make even the bare minimum payments on our credit card bills. My continued use of new, low interest credit accounts, allowed me to pay down balances on old accounts. I was managing month by month, not wanting to look at the big picture, but I knew it was a juggling act that was not sustainable. Sometime soon, one of the juggled balls was bound to drop.

Sharon and Doug, aware of my situation, suggested we meet with their accountant to get his advice. Laying it all out before him, seeing it through another's eyes, confirmed what I already knew but had been somehow been keeping at arm's length. We were in dire straits. There was talk of bankruptcy. There was talk of "walking away" from the house. There was talk of protecting retirement fund assets. I had never once in my whole life not paid a debt. The idea of walking away from the house was repugnant to me. Bankruptcy was repugnant. I was 74. I'd worked hard all of my life. We'd set money aside for the nest egg that, over the course of the past year, I'd watched shrink from turkey-sized to hen-sized. My head was spinning.

In the meantime, I was pulling soaking wet towels from the linen closet and putting them back in the dryer. Hiding laundry soap in an attempt to keep Mike from doing a whole load with only one or two pieces in it. He'd always done more than his share of the laundry, and of the two of us he was the neatest when it came to folding things and putting them away. I didn't want him to be at a loss for any of his usual routines, but I was on constant damage control duty.

I was also on constant damage control duty with our finances. Which card could I draw money from to make the payments for whatever month's bills I was looking at? Would I have to pull money from an IRA account to make ends meet? Even with the bursting of the real estate bubble, we still had some equity in our house. In the past, home equity had provided a sense of security, but the recent bursting of the real estate bubble changed things. How much? I wondered. I set up an appointment with Joanie B., the real estate agent who had handled the sale of our first Gold River home and the purchase of the home we were now in. Next I arranged for a friend to take Mike to a movie on the afternoon of Joanie's visit.

We sat sipping tea in the living room while I told her of my dilemma, and she told me of hers. She'd heard from a neighbor that Mike was having cognitive difficulties, but hadn't known to what extent. I'd heard of the real estate crash, but hadn't known to what extent.

"The market's totally tanked," she said. "I haven't sold a house in two months. No one in our office has. Luckily Jim's job seems fairly secure, but I don't know what we'd do without his paycheck."

As with others of my generation, I grew up with the mostly unspoken but powerful taboo against talking about sex or money. I took a deep breath and plunged rapid-fire into the forbidden territory of money.

"We're in a mess. Mike can't function either as a choir director or as a professional singer. My once healthy book sales are practically nil. School budgets have been slashed. Teachers and librarians have no money for supplemental reading material. There's no education money available for staff development workshops or author visits to schools, so no more of that. I'm nearly as unemployable as Mike is. Really, we should be able to live on our teachers' retirement funds, but our expenses are over the top. In 2007 our combined musician/writer income, beyond our retirement income, was around $30,000. This year we'll be lucky to hit $1,000. I've always thought that if things got too tight, we could sell the house … "

"How much do you owe?"

"Around $230,000."

"Even if you could sell this house, which I doubt, you wouldn't clear enough to cover costs. Seller fees, repairs—you'd probably have to replace the fence. All of the fences in here have passed their use-by date. I haven't seen one recently that's not full of dry rot. It would end up costing you money to sell," Joanie said.

I sat stunned for a moment. It was bad news that we would get nothing from the sale of our house. Worse news that it would actually cost us money to sell it. But I trusted Joanie's real estate smarts.

"I can't stay here," I told her. "I can't manage the maintenance on my own. Mike goes from room to room looking for things, moving things around. I just get one room put back together and he's been through two more. Plus I can't really afford the monthly payments or the HOA fees."

Joanie gave me a long, slow look. Speaking in a near whisper, she said, "You didn't hear this from me. Understand? What I'm about to say, I didn't say."

I nodded in puzzled agreement.

"What some people might do, have done in similar situations, is stop making their house payments. That frees up money for other bills. It's taking banks up to a year to actually foreclose. Longer sometimes. Free rent for a year."

I gazed out the sliding glass doors that led to the patio. I watched the water in the fountain of Mike's handiwork steadily bubbling.

"I don't think I can bring myself to do that."

"You might be surprised. I'm just sayin'…. Remember how we celebrated when we closed the deal on this house? It's a great house," Joanie said, looking around the living room and out onto the patio. "Great floor plan. I sort of wanted it myself."

"It could still be yours," I told her.

She laughed—not that full-out kind of laugh that erupts when something's funny. More the subdued half-laugh that recognizes irony, or futility, or the general trials of life.

Joanie stood to leave. I walked with her to the door. Before she stepped outside she turned to face me. "Think about what I didn't say. Think about what you didn't hear from me. Everybody's in a mess. You're not the only one."

We hugged goodbye and I watched as she walked down the pathway to her car. We would not be celebrating.

September 13, 2016

Dear Mike,

You would want to know that I'm okay. I am okay. Really, I'm better than okay. I'm writing this to you today, from Martha's Vineyard, on my 81st birthday. Here for two weeks on a writing workshop/retreat at the Noepe Center for Literary Arts, I am breathing the crisp, pure air of the island, writing from morning into the early afternoon, walking the town, the cemetery, the beach, sharing meals and conversation with my fellow writers. My hope is to soon finish this account of our difficult FTD years and get back to fiction. Fiction will be more fun, but I'm dedicated to first getting this story out into the world.

When I leave here, I'll go home to a little duplex in River Park, on a corner lot with a big, wide lawn and four huge elm-like shade trees. Zelkovas, they're called. From the time I first noticed the "For Rent" sign on this duplex, I lusted after the trees. Then when I met the landlord there for an inside look, I lusted after the whole place. I'd been living in an okay duplex just a few blocks over, but it was a bit dark. To get to the backyard I had to walk down three treacherous, not-to-code steps and through the garage. It was okay for me—there was a grab bar, and I was used to maneuvering the steps. I sometimes found myself holding my breath, though, as one of my contemporaries made her way down the steps and out to the patio. The laundry was in the garage. The carpeting was less than pristine. Still it was a definite step up from my nomading days, and, unlike that first apartment, it had a spacious yard for Sunny.

Because money had been so tight, I spent a sleepless night stewing over whether or not I could afford to move. If I did, I would be leaving the first place a month before my lease was up. Plus, the corner place was $200 more a month than I'd been paying.

In the morning I crunched numbers. It was a stretch, and nothing a wise financial adviser would have encouraged. But no place had felt like home since we'd left Gold River. This place, with its gleaming hardwood floors, a large living room window and back door slider that provided dawn to dusk natural light, a freshly updated kitchen, a small but nicely landscaped patio—this place could feel like home. I took the leap and emailed my application to the owner first thing that morning. He—we'll call him Frank—had several applications. Although I still had the black mark of bankruptcy on my credit report, I also had three recent years of consistent, on time, rent payment records.

After the application, I emailed a letter to Frank, telling him I was the very best choice of a tenant he could ever have. Nearly all of my life I'd lived in houses I'd owned. I still treated a house as if it were my own. I was old and single. No raucous parties for me. I had no pets. I don't remember what else I said, but I won the toss.

It's a pretty little two-bedroom place, or in my case, one-bedroom, one-office place. The patio outside the kitchen sliders has no treacherous steps to maneuver to get there. A number of plants in large, colorful pots add color to the outdoor space. A table for six, sometimes pushed to seat eight, is a nice gathering place on a Delta breeze-infused, cool Sacramento evening. In the living room is a fireplace with a mantel; there's a convenient breakfast bar in the kitchen, and plenty of natural light. As my heart knew the first time I stepped inside, it feels like home.

Ten years ago, before FTD hit, before the recession hit, sitting at my home office writing desk, the 5-by-4-foot teak desk, three walls lined, floor to ceiling, with oak book-shelves, gazing out the window onto the redwood lined pathway that wound throughout the so-called village, the path that we so often followed, grandkids running in front of us to get to the pool and an afternoon of swimming, or that we followed in the other direction to parties at the Taylors', or the Richmonds'—from that vantage point I could not have foretold life as I now live it.

These days, when I pause in whatever it is I'm doing, working on some writing project, say this one, or checking email, or Facebook, or spiraling along on one of those one-thing-leads-to-another wild goose Google chases, I gaze through my office corner windows onto a different walkway, one that leads directly to a sidewalk where I might see the 3- and 5-year-old neighbor kids zipping along on their twin scooters. Or any manner of dogs out walking their owners. Rarely, an owner may be walking a dog, but it's usually the other way around, the way Sunny used to walk us.

I'm doing a bit of part-time teaching at the county Youth Detention Facility. The schedule is easy and the work, though challenging, is, I feel, important. The paycheck is welcome.

I recently led a staff development workshop in New Mexico, and a few months back I did an author visit to a school in Fresno. That business may be picking up now that the worst of the recession is over. A little more earned income, coupled with much lower expenses now that there's only one of me to support, means the financial strain has somewhat eased. I still have to watch my dollars, but I no longer have to count each penny.

Mornings when I wake up in what is now my home, the first thing I do (well … the second thing I do) is open the blinds and curtains and greet the day. Sometimes I go for a morning walk or go to the gym. Too often I go right to my computer and sit too long.

I miss you in the mornings, shared coffee and newspaper, your intermittent questions of "what's a five-letter word for … ?" Our sharing of expectations for the day. Or maybe there was talk of whatever book we were reading, or what movies we wanted to see, or talk of our kids, our grandkids, conversations that don't really work with anyone else. So, yes, I still miss you.

Unlike what I hear from my newly single contemporaries, our old friends, couples, often include me in dinners, out or in, and still seem happy to do things with me. I'm aware it's mostly a couples' world, especially for our generation. And I also suspect that I'm not as interesting in a group, alone, as I was with you.

A year or so back I was at a brunch, three married couples and me. The couples were telling stories of each other's foibles, not in that nasty "Who's Afraid of Virginia Woolf" way, but with a light-heartedness, a generosity of spirit that seemed to preclude any hurt or embarrassment that can sometimes come with such tales.

The youngest couple's wife joked about how she was always trying to get Jerry out for walks. He would reluctantly agree to a walk but then would drag his feet to the extent that his heart rate might be even slower than when he was on the couch watching TV. But when they finally turned to go home, he picked up his pace, like an old nag headed back to the stables.

"Because I'm walking behind you and watching your butt. Because I have hopes for when we get home," Jerry explained.

The husband of one of the more mature couples told of snorkeling in Hawaii and after 15 minutes or so of being stunned by the beauty of the underwater scene, he saw floating, just off to his left, a $100 bill. He grabbed it and sure enough it was the real thing. Then he noticed another and another. Maybe they would go to that highly touted, expensive restaurant for dinner that night after all. He collected five $100 bills until they stopped coming. He hurried up to the beach where his wife was sitting.

"Look! Look what I just found floating in the water! Five $100 bills!"

He said she gave him a long look, the kind she often gives when he's done something ridiculously stupid.

"What?" he said.

"How much money did you have in the pocket of your trunks?"

He reached into his pocket, only to find emptiness where, before they left the condominium, he had placed five $100 bills.

I mentioned this to Donna and Dennis when we met for the once-a-year dinner we share when they drive up from San Gabriel to spend a week or two with their daughter in Vallejo. I mentioned that I may not be nearly as much fun without you than I was with you.

"Well …," Donna said, "we did love the Mike and Marilyn show." They went on to assure me that I was still absolutely fascinating, but I thought they were at least half lying.

On the way back from that dinner, where Donna and Dennis had shared a few of their own amusing couples stories, I considered my dilemma. I didn't really want to couple up with anyone, not that eligible couplers have been beating down my door. I've been on a total of three dates in the past three years, and although the men were all nice people, I was bored. You were, when you were you, never boring. I didn't want to go out for another of those dinners, and I certainly wasn't interested in crawling into bed with any of them. That part of me may be closed for the duration. I'm not sure. That remains to be seen.

In answer to my solo dullness, I conjured an imaginary lover. His name is Mario McCarthy—some Latin passion coupled with Irish humor. He's a good choice. Sometimes I take him to dinner with me. I tell stories about him, about his foibles and our escapades. I don't introduce him to everyone. Some people are still offended by mixed marriages. You know, one of us is real, the other is not.

We've chosen not to live together. I don't want to have to argue with him over home decor and I'm afraid his taste might be similar to yours. Anyway, Mario is part of my okayness.

I'm in good health as are all of our kids and grandkids. I have meaningful work, good friends, and am, finally, financially stable again. I'm more and more aware that each day brings me closer to the end. That's always been the case, for all of us, but at 81, the balance has shifted. The days have become more precious. Although I wish we were sharing them, I wake up every morning, grateful for the gift of the day ahead of me.

I'm now more of a regular, productive member of UUSS than I have been for some time. I appreciate the structure that offers opportunities to take some positive action in the world—welcoming refugees, fighting racism, offering support for homeless families…. I also appreciate the Sunday services that pull me out of my little life and into a broader world view. I don't do nearly as much as I might, but I do more than I would if I were not a part of that organization.

My books, the ones in the Hamilton High Series, have a new publisher, New Wind Publishing. It was one of those serendipitous meetings in which things come together in an almost magical way. I'm so glad the books are still in print. In their own small way, they sometimes do some good in the world. So that, too, is part of my okayness.

What else would you want to be reassured of? I may not be dressing according to your tastes, but that's no surprise, is it? I don't see Ashley or Kerry as often as we once did, but that's just the nature of things. What else?

If you were sitting across from me now, over a cup of coffee, or a glass of wine, I think your mind would be put to rest that I am doing fine. There will be at least one more hard time to come. I know that. But for now, the hardest of the hard times are over and life, for me, is good.

Marilyn

OUR LAST GOLD RIVER CHRISTMAS

December 2009

Mike had always been Mr. Christmas, weaving glittery garlands along the stairway banister, draping them around the mirror over the fireplace, outlining the windows with garlands. Garlands everywhere. He arranged the 12 chorister figures, including the little dog in the Santa hat and the boy with a French horn, on the bar in the living room. A wreath at the front door and another over the fireplace. Traditionally we chose a tree together, but Mike was always the decorator. Over the years he'd collected Christmas ornaments from our travels—Germany, England, Vienna, Scotland. There were also whimsical ornaments, a "Wizard of Oz" tin man, and Dorothy. There was a stuffed fat ballerina in leotards, a sparkly Peter Pan, and the treasured ornaments for each grandchild.

On Christmas Eve, Mike was always the one who handed out the presents, waiting for each person to unwrap and exclaim over the gift before going on to the next. He started with the youngest, then moved on in order of age until Aunt Hazel, in her 80s, had her turn. Then he would start over again.

"Oh, look! Here's one for Kerry from the Wicked Witch of the West!"

"Here's one for Subei from Rudolph!"

Traditionally he wrapped and labeled the presents. To Ashley from the Tooth Fairy. To Marilyn from Mr. Claus.

I did some of the shopping for gifts, though mostly Mike and I gift shopped together. The annual letter was my doing. I prepared the house for our family overnighters and did most of the grocery shopping. Making the Christmas lasagna was usually a joint project, though sometimes I got solo lasagna duty. But really? All of the trappings of Christmas were Mike's. Every aspect of Christmas was Mike-infused.

Back in 2009, just after the first of December, Mike retrieved box after box of decorations from the attic and schlepped them downstairs. When I wandered into the living room with a draft of our holiday letter to run past him, he was dragging lights and garland out of two boxes and piling them on the couch.

"How're you doing?" I asked.

"Fine," he said, not looking up as he straightened out a long strand of blue garland.

"I think I've finally finished our letter. Can I read it to you?"

"Of course."

He still didn't look up.

I started, "2009 was filled with …"

"We need more garland."

"Okay, but Mike, can you listen to our letter? Let me know what you think?"

He glanced my way. "Sure, I can do that."

"2009 was a year filled with endings and beginnings …"

Mike walked out of the room, went into my office and started rummaging through the desk. "Where are the thumbtacks?"

I started the silent "Ode to Joy" chant, "It's not his fault. It's not his fault. It's not his fault, no, it's not." and found the thumbtacks for him.

By lunchtime, Mike had emptied all of the boxes, the contents of which were strewn all over the living room, on the couch, chairs, bar, floor. In addition to the overabundance of accumulated Christmas decorations, there was a large ceramic Easter bunny, a spring wreath, ceramic Halloween jack-o-lanterns, a whimsical witch poised on her broomstick, and other tchotchkes. I managed to repack and put away a few out-of-season items while Mike was struggling to get a string of outdoor lights up and working around a patio trellis. He was beyond the point of moving from Step A to Step B if Step A wasn't working, and he soon gave up on the trellis lights. In addition to mismatched garlands, a tree with ornaments huddled in a few places and bare in others, there was the Easter bunny, the jack-o-lanterns, and the witch, items I'd not been fast enough to pack away and move out of the living room when I repacked other autumn, spring, summer items. It didn't matter. None of that mattered.

We were all determined to keep things as normal as possible for Mike. On Christmas Eve he sat beside the tree and began distributing gifts. He handed them out as quickly as possible, one after the other, until the kids were overwhelmed with the piles in front of them, opening one quickly, setting it aside, going on to the next. Even though I'd made sure the "To" labels were clear and accurate, several gifts reached the wrong hands. Mike handed 3-year-old Mika a small, nicely wrapped box, which she opened eagerly. Inside was a pair of earrings. Mika loved, still loves, all things sparkly, and she was quite pleased with her gift.

"Oh, those are for Gramma," Mike said, reaching to take the package from her.

She clutched the package in both hands and hung on, looking to be on the verge of tears.

I suggested Mike find another package for Mika. There were plenty.

I moved over beside Mika.

"Your earrings are beautiful," I said. "May I see them again?"

She loosened her grip to give me a peek. In the meantime, Mike was again racing to get packages dispersed. I pointed out that the earrings were for pierced ears. She readily agreed to let me keep them safe for her until she got her ears pierced. She even allowed as how I might wear them on special occasions.

On Christmas morning, Mike made a big pot of coffee as he always did. Except that he'd put in coffee for two cups and water for 12. One by one, people quietly walked to the sink and poured their coffee out. He was at a point where as soon as he started one thing he was eager, even anxious, to go on to the next.

"Shall I put the lasagna in now?" he asked.

"Let's wait until around 3," I said. "It's only 10 now," as if telling him the time would make a difference.

"Oh, okay," he said, walking to the refrigerator and taking out the lasagna.

Sharon asked if Mike wanted to take Sunny for a walk with her and Enzo, their big, gentle, moose of a dog.

"Sure," he said, getting Sunny's leash.

I put the lasagna away.

Mike was back with Sunny within minutes. Once out, he needed to get back home.

Late that afternoon, before we sat down to dinner, Mike got the martini shaker from the living room bar. He didn't drink martinis, but those of us who did appreciated his expertise. However, remembering the morning coffee, I told

Sharon I thought maybe we should ask Dale to mix up the martinis.

"I think Dad needs to do what he always does."

She was right, of course. Mike filled the shaker and did his martini-shaking dance to the rhythm of "La Cucaracha," then poured the icy mixture into the glasses he loved so much he once tried to become a martini drinker.

After the toast and the first overwhelming sip of what might have been straight vermouth, martinis sat on kitchen counters and family room side tables, and I poured the wine.

Mike had set the table early in the day. As always, he'd used his Aunt Ursie's white linen tablecloth, the one he'd had washed with special care at a French Hand Laundry. But unlike earlier Christmases, the table was set with a hodgepodge of dishes, some of his family china, some Christmas dishes. The silverware, too, was hodgepodge, all sadly symbolic of the increasing hodgepodge of Mike's brain.

I shifted a few things around, making sure that every setting had a knife and fork, and let the rest go. Matching china patterns, placements of utensils, napkins on the "right" side of the plates—none of that was consequential.

Mike sat at the head of the table and served the Christmas lasagna. He served sausage lasagna to the vegetarians, vegetable lasagna to the carnivores, but that was an easy fix. Mike ate quickly, not joining the conversation. When he was finished, he carried his plate to the kitchen, then came back to clear the table. "Not yet," first one and then another laughed as they guarded their unfinished dinners.

"Shall I get the cake?" Mike asked.

Stalling for time, I walked him to the kitchen where the very fancy cake still sat in its bakery box. "Can you get the cake cutter?"

"Sure," he said, and went to the china cabinet and took the cake cutter from the drawer.

"How about the cake plate?"

Again he went to the cabinet and brought out the cake plate.

"Shall we make coffee?"

"Sure."

He filled the coffee pot with water, put the filter in top, and put in two heaping tablespoons of coffee. I added more coffee as Mike took the cake from the box.

Mike cleared the table of dinner plates and brought in the cake. Unlike most Christmases, no one overindulged with second helpings of lasagna in 2009. They were lucky to have finished one helping.

We sang "Happy Birthday" to Dale, Mike served the cake, poured the coffee, finished his dessert quickly, took his cup and plate to the kitchen, and came back to clear the table. He hovered until one by one people finished and gave up their dessert plates. I followed him into the kitchen and put the dessert plates into the dishwasher as he rinsed them. He'd already loaded up the dinner plates. When the last dessert plate was placed in the rack, Mike announced he was going to bed.

"It's a little early," I told him.

"I'm going to bed."

He stood in the hall outside the dining room and said, "Goodnight. I'm going to bed."

People called their thanks out to him as he climbed the stairs.

By this time the kids were playing with their gifts, or watching TV. The adults lingered at the table, sad and drained.

We bemoaned the fact that so far no anti-anxiety meds had eased Mike's agitation. We tried to guess at the next progression. Hazel said over and over, "I just don't know why this had to happen to such a nice man. Mike was always such a nice man."

I knew without a doubt that this was the last time we would all be seated around this table that had for decades held so much food for so many of us.

When the house payment came due on the first of January, I didn't take the mortgage coupon from its special little box. I didn't take my checkbook from the drawer. I didn't make a house payment. Not then, nor the next month, nor the next.

THE DREADED
DRIVING DECISION
January through April 2010

I agonized over Mike's driving. Not long after driving the rental car at night with no lights on, Mike made a trip to the library to return books, then came back, books in hand, saying the library wasn't there anymore. The library was not far from home, and was a very familiar place to Mike.

Soon I was driving wherever we went that was unfamiliar, or more than a few miles, though Mike continued to drive to our local market, and to Camerata rehearsals, which were just a few miles from home. Friends and family now often asked, "Is Mike/Dad still driving?" I knew the implied question: "Why is Mike/Dad still driving?"

In my heart of hearts, I knew Mike shouldn't be driving, but I dreaded the time when I would have to take him everywhere, and when I wouldn't even have one of those brief respites to myself, when he was at the market, or at the local Starbucks. Finally, though, good sense won out. One morning, while he was showering, I called Dr. Carlson and asked that she notify the DMV that Mike suffered from dementia and should no longer be driving.

In February 2010, the "order of suspension/revocation" notice from the DMV showed up in our mailbox. Mike showed little response to the news. I assured him I would take him wherever he needed to go, and that was the end of it until a few mornings later when he wanted to drive to the market.

"I'll take you," I said.

"No! I'll drive myself!"

I showed him the DMV notice that was still sitting on the table next to the telephone.

"You can't drive now, hon. I'll be your chauffeur," I told him.

He went to the phone and called the doctor. Surprisingly, he got through to her. He asked that she call the DMV and tell them he could drive. She said that she couldn't do that. He hung up and went upstairs to bed. When I went to check on him half an hour or so later, he turned to look at me. "I've always been able to drive," he said.

I sat beside him on the bed, rubbing his back and shoulders.

"I'm sorry things are so hard for you these days. But I can help. I love you. I'll help."

He rolled to the other side of the bed, threw the covers back and got up.

"I've always been able to drive!"

Later the next week, Corry's family and friends gathered in Berkeley to celebrate her completion of a master's degree in history. She'd managed this after years of juggling classes and study time with a full-time workload, so it was definitely time to party. I drove us over in the Honda, telling Mike we were going to leave the car with Doug, who would take it to a place he knew to get it detailed. This much was true. What I didn't say was that the same auto-detailing place, as prearranged with Doug, would be putting the car on their sales lot.

The party was great fun. Mike and I danced for a few songs, then he went on to dance with several of the other women, all longtime friends. It was if, for a few hours, the old Mike was back. While he was on the dance floor, I slipped the Honda keys and pink slip to Doug. We rode back to Sacramento with Dale and Marg.

In the morning Mike piled up the week's newspapers and took them to the recycling container in the garage. He was back in an instant.

"Where's my car??"

I reminded him that Doug was taking it in for detailing work. I confessed that we would be leaving it over there to be sold. Mike went upstairs to bed.

If I were to rank the decision to have Mike's license revoked on a scale of one to 10, I'd think it was about a seven. The decision to move us to a retirement community: a 10. Squared. I was convinced of the need to be proactive, but maybe we could hang on in Gold River for a while longer? If Joanie's estimate was correct, we had at least another eight months before the actual foreclosure.

Shortly after the Riverside visit, I was felled by a nasty cold/flu bug that had been making the rounds. Most of the day I'd been in our upstairs bedroom, bundled in throws and a comforter, stretched out on the chaise. So much to do and there I was, not making phone calls, or doing any of the much needed organizing of my office, the one place I could purge without much interference from Mike.

The good news about this very minor illness was that it removed any lurking doubts about the wisdom of the moving decision. That morning in bed, sore throat, fever, achy, I asked Mike if he would call our dentist's office to cancel my 10 o'clock appointment. "Sure," he said. "Is the number in my book?" I said it was. I also asked if he'd take Sunny out. "Sure," he said, not moving. Sunny increased her whining, scratching, let-me-out behavior. "Could you take her out now?" I asked. "Sure," he said, still lying there.

"When?"

"Right now!"

But he didn't move. I got up and took care of the necessities. The shortest possible walk with Sunny had me shivering with chills on my return. I dragged myself back to the chaise. I couldn't help thinking, though, about how that would have been had I really been sick.

I gave Mike his meds, which he could no longer manage on his own, and reminded him to eat a bite—he could fix a bowl of cereal with sliced banana, but he had to be reminded. I had to admit that it would be good to be at a place where meals were provided and, if needed, help would be available.

For the rest of the day I popped aspirin and dozed. At 6, Mike was downstairs watching CNN. He was scheduled to be picked up for a Camerata rehearsal in 15 minutes. I went downstairs and put the after-rehearsal wine it was his turn to take in a bag and reminded him to take it. I'd done nothing about dinner for us, but one missed dinner was no disaster.

Back to the chaise.

Afternoon two of the nasty bug had me searching through the refrigerator in hope that dinner would magically appear. I saw that between a chunk of leftover rice from Thai food takeout, and some hunks of beef in the freezer, I almost had the ingredients for a quick beef stroganoff dish.

"Would you mind picking up a few things at Bel Air?" I asked Mike.

"I can do that," he said, turning away from the ever-looping "A Streetcar Named Desire."

I made a list, knowing even in the cold/flu fog that five things were a lot, but forging ahead. I read the list to Mike: medium-sized sour cream, a head of lettuce, cherry tomatoes, orange juice, a package of mushrooms from the produce department.

"Do you have money?"

He took his wallet from his back pocket and counted out $26.

"Plenty," I told him.

"Where are the keys?" he asked.

"No, hon, you'll have to walk."

He looked at me blankly.

"Your license isn't valid. You'll have to walk. Or maybe I should just drive you over later."

"No, I can walk!" he said, irritated. "I know how to do that!"

Bel Air was five blocks away. The weather was nice. It was good for Mike to get out and about. These were all things I reminded myself of as he stomped out the door.

Twenty minutes later, Mike was back, happy, eating from a large Yogurt Monkey container.

"Mint," he said, smiling. "I got everything."

"Everything" consisted of a small container of strawberry flavored cream cheese, orange juice, lamb chops, a dozen eggs (we already had an untouched carton of eggs in the refrigerator), and bananas.

"No sour cream?"

"Oh. Didn't I do the right thing?" he asked, the turned-up corners of his smile turning downward.

"No. It's fine. We need sour cream for stroganoff, but we can have something else."

"I can go back."

"No, we'll find plenty to eat."

"No, I'll go back."

"Well ... if you feel like it."

"Sure. Where are the keys?"

"Well ... you'll need to walk."

"Okay! Okay! I can do that!"

He was back soon, finishing another large Yogurt Monkey, unloading a quart container of chocolate chip ice cream, a large package of cream cheese, cherry tomatoes and Chinese cabbage.

"Okay?" he said.

"Great. Thank you for doing that," I said, smiling. That should have been my response to his *first* return from the store, but it took me a while to figure that out.

He settled back to "A Streetcar Named Desire," and I threw something together that I loosely called dinner. We finished it off with mounds of ice cream.

In the morning I called Riverside and arranged to put a $500 hold on the downstairs apartment with the little patio. I'd done the math. I figured I could keep us there for at least a year and a half, maybe two, before every retirement account was drained, and we'd reach rock bottom. It was a frightening situation. But, I reminded myself, it was nothing in comparison to what post-earthquake displaced Haitians were experiencing, or what any of the estimated 100,000 homeless Iraqis had to deal with, or, for that matter, what the growing number of homeless people here in Sacramento went through every day.

A 6-BY-5-FOOT
AQUARIUM

Spring 2010

Because of Mike's diagnosis, the director of Riverside's memory care program needed to evaluate his condition before we could be accepted into an independent living space. Rachel Martin came to our house for the evaluation. She was lively and charming and soon won Mike's confidence. His other neuropsychological evaluations took place in offices where he was uncomfortable and prone to defensiveness, but he was relaxed at home with Rachel. I felt her evaluation offered a much more accurate version of what was up with Mike than any of the previous evaluations. They laughed and talked easily during the course of her two hours with him.

As she was leaving, Rachel handed me her card with three phone numbers—work, home and cell—and her email address.

"I'm yours for life," she said. "Once I've evaluated someone, they're always part of my caseload."

Later that day, Rachel emailed me a copy of the results that she would pass on to Carolyn. Nothing in her report surprised me, but it was striking to see it all listed in this form:

- Subject answers questions or performs tasks without realizing the consequences of his actions.
- Difficulty learning and retaining new information.
- Difficulty comprehending logic.
- Difficulty initiating a new activity outside of his routine.
- Difficulty with impatience.
- Difficulty sequencing daily activities.
- Beginning to have difficulty identifying common objects visually; however, if the object is described he can identify it.
- Periods of delusion, takes events in his life and mixes them up with other events. May say things like, "I throw stones at squirrels to keep them from

eating the hummingbirds"; however, in reality he does not throw stones at squirrels and, due to his inability to comprehend logic, if you tell him that squirrels are vegetarians, he becomes confrontational.

- Difficulty with calculations and numbers.
- Difficulty with time relationships.
- Wants to please.
- Denial of any memory difficulties or medical problems.
- Flight of ideas when in a conversation.
- Requires routine and structure to prevent heightened anxiety.
- Difficulty with comprehension.
- May have difficulty telling family or care providers if he has pain, however he will act out and have a change of behavior.
- Difficulty when confronted due to lack of comprehension of logic.
- Mild OCD tendencies.

Carolyn called the day after the evaluation to say that although Mike's condition would generally disqualify us from entering the independent living section, both she and Rachel were convinced that, because of my competence and attitude, we'd do fine there. It was reassuring to learn that two objective observers considered me to be competent. I wasn't feeling so competent right then.

I visited Riverside again for the purpose of checking out the apartment I'd reserved. I got a floor plan complete with measurements. The total living space was about 500 square feet. I tried to picture us living there. I got scared. It was simply too tiny. It was too expensive. Carolyn returned my deposit check, and I continued the hunt.

The "Gentle Breeze" place with three goldfish swimming around in a bowl on the front counter was most affordable, but we weren't yet at rock bottom, and that's what it would have taken for me to move us into such a place. The staff, probably overworked and underpaid, was unfriendly. Residents aimlessly walked the hallways or were parked against a wall, strapped into wheelchairs, probably overmedicated. It would not be winning any awards for cleanliness.

I finally settled on a 6-foot-by-5-foot aquarium place, Carmichael Oaks, only a few miles from our Gold River house. It was slightly less expensive than Riverside, and it had the great advantage of comparatively spacious apartments.

Though downsizing from a 2,700-square-foot residence to a 1,000-square-foot apartment still presented a daunting task, it did look like a space we could live in. The marketing director there, Charlotte, and the executive director, Janice, were both charming and accommodating. They moved the upright piano from the lobby/living room down to the assisted living wing, making room for Mike's beloved Mason & Hamlin baby grand.

When I asked if we could paint one of the walls in our apartment living room with an accent color, they said sure. Provide the paint, and Marco, the maintenance man, would paint it for us. Marco! He painted the wall and put organizers in our closet. He set up the solar-powered water fountain Dale and I had chosen for our balcony. He was there within minutes when the toilet became clogged. Maybe retirement home living wouldn't be so bad after all.

August 2015

Dear Mike,

I put clean sheets on the bed today. Not our king-sized, solid oak, Craftsman-style Stickley bed. The one we shared for such a long, long time. The one that held laughter and tears, love and passion. Not that one. That one was sold through a consignment store. That one was too big for my scaled-down life.

I put the freshly washed, basic full-sized cotton sheet set, bought at Penney's when I moved into the little duplex, on the new, basic bed. They're serviceable—not as soft as the sage green, 800-thread-count, Egyptian cotton sheets that were last on our old bed. I remember when you brought those sheets home.

"They were on sale," you said, as if "on sale" was the same thing as "free," or even "affordable."

How you loved new sheets and new towels. Even with the abundant closet and cupboard space in our Gold River house, the linen closets were bulging with sheets, and towels, and tablecloths. Like your sock drawer, you kept our linen closets beautifully organized. Did you know how much I appreciated that organization? Did I ever tell you? I hope so.

I think of you every time I open my linen closet here in River Park. Things are bunched up, not ever-so-neatly folded and stacked. Yesterday I opened a cupboard door and a bath towel fell out. You would have laughed at me, then re-folded the contents of the cupboard. I laugh at me, too, but I don't re-fold. It's not my nature the way it was in yours.

By the time I pull the contour sheet over the fourth corner, you are there. I see you wrestling the bottom sheet over the fourth corner of our California King mattress, then pulling it taut, all corners even. As I tuck the top sheet under the foot of the basic mattress, I see you, forming a tight, perfect fold at each end of the foot of the mattress, then carefully folding the soft, sage green top over our favorite wool blanket, fluffing the comforter, arranging the freshly cased pillows, the end product worthy of a magazine cover.

You couldn't stand a loose top sheet. On the rare occasion when one of your corners didn't hold, when one of us had somehow kicked the top sheet loose, you would get up, even in the middle of the night, and redo the loose corner.

Back in the days when grief and loss seemed so far away that we could laugh at the possibilities, we would joke that if I someday woke to find you lying cold and dead beside me, all I would need to do would be to kick the top sheet loose and you would rise and fix it. If things were reversed, you could drag my lifeless body to the shower, prop me up under the steamy flow of hot water, and I would slowly revive, as I revived every day with my early morning shower.

I finish making the bed, knowing that within a night or two the top sheet will come loose. I won't fix it. I don't mind a rumpled bed. I'd rather be sitting here, writing to you, than remaking a bed. And no matter how tightly I fitted the corners, or how carefully I tucked in the bottom sheet, it would still not be our bed. Our bed is a thing of the past.

Here's the thing, though. No matter how I try to change my sleeping position to the left side of the bed, or even the middle, I always wake up on the right side. My head knows the days of our sharing a bed are over. My heart knows it, too. But it's as if my body hasn't caught up. As if my sound-asleep body moves to the right, expecting you to come in late from a rehearsal, or a performance, and slide into your side of the bed, silently curling your body close to mine.

I visited you at Sister Sarah's yesterday. Until several weeks ago you would smile and give me a hug when I walked in, or when I met you outside as you were walking your loop. Both the smile and the hug were glancing, a millisecond interruption in your determined path. But since I've started bringing cookies each time I visit, you reach for my hand, focused only on the baggy of cookies. Four. Chocolate chip. That's what I bring to you. I buy them in bulk from Raley's and keep them frozen, removing four at a time, knowing they'll be thawed by the time I get to Orangevale.

It's interesting to me that you remember that. It's a set routine for you. Also interesting that you always reach for my right hand. Even if I keep both hands behind me so that the cookies can't be seen, it's the right hand you choose. If I stopped bringing cookies, how long would it take for you to forget that routine and go back to giving me a quick hug? But I won't try that experiment. There is so little left for you to enjoy, and the cookies bring you some brief moments of joy.

I wish I could talk directly to you, but you're constantly on the move. When I walk beside you, it is not a companionable walk—it's just me following along with you totally focused on the next step, and the next.

How much speech can you understand? When Sang or Daniel say, "Michael. Give me a hug!" you open your arms. When the doctor asks that you take a big breath, you do. Always when I visit, you go to the parked Prius and try the door on the passenger side. It's always locked. That's a habit from before, back when you were angry and unmanageable. I was afraid you'd get in the car, and we'd not be able to get you out. But you're cooperative now. When you try to open the door, I tell you, "We're not going anywhere today," and you walk on.

What if you still understand speech even though you can't initiate it?

I could try taking you for a ride again. Have you in a confined place so I could talk to you. I want to tell you how much I've enjoyed most of our years together. How much I've loved you. How I'm doing as right by you as I possibly can. You're okay in the car now, as far as safety goes. But once out of the driveway, you're anxious. You sit, body tense, leaning forward, looking straight ahead, eager, I think, to get back "home." I become anxious, too. Nothing is easy.

Goodbye for now. You are always, always, in my heart. I'll see you in a few days, cookies in hand.

Marilyn

THE TABLE
April 2010

Early in the morning, I put Mike on a plane to Burbank, where he was met by Anne and Bob, longtime friends. They walked the streets of Pasadena, eating at restaurants he'd loved from our Altadena days. They browsed Vroman's bookstore, the oldest and largest independent bookstore in Southern California. They stopped in at one of Anne and Mike's all-time favorite places, Jacob Maarse, described on their website as "the gold standard in floral innovation, craftsmanship and aesthetic refinement." They kept him busy, busy, busy, then sent him back to Sacramento the next evening. During that time I was free to pick up moving boxes, take them to a new storage unit, make a myriad of sensitive phone calls, and revisit our new dwelling place at Carmichael Oaks.

The morning I returned from taking Mike to the airport, I sat at the dining room table, going over my lengthy, pre-move to-do list—cancel automatic deposits in preparation for switching checking accounts, arrange times and details with movers, get yet another detail of the power of attorney transfer notarized, call Southwest to be sure I can escort Mike to the gate and wait with him until boarding time when he flies to Florida next month. Get TB tests required for Carmichael Oaks entrance, get "soiree" on the Carmichael Oaks calendar, assess non-liquid assets, work on the next chapter of *Over 70 and I Don't Mean Miles Per Hour*, get contract to Hiram Johnson High School for coming school visit, take the car to be serviced … I had so many lists, and folders, and telephone messages that I'd moved my computer away from my cluttered desk and into the dining room, expanding the clutter onto the dining room table.

I stared absent-mindedly at the teak table as I sipped coffee and pondered which of the many tasks that lay before me I should start with. A light scratch in the table caught my attention. I remembered when we bought the table at the Pasadena Plummers store, more than 35 years ago—the table that's had all those Christmases worth of both meat and vegetable lasagna, Caesar salads, and grandiose Christmas/birthday cakes for Dale. It's the table around which my mother, and Mike's Aunt Virginia and Uncle Norman, and Marg's mother, Thelma, and Norman's second wife, Jean, and Mike's parents, and my Aunt Gladys, and so many others of the dearly and not-so-dearly departed gathered, Christmas after Christmas, as if the Christmas gatherings around the Danish teak table would go on and on and on. And it's not only remnants of the departed captured in the patina of the table. There's the resonance of the still living hovering just below the surface of the now worn teak—laughter, complaints, talk of politics and the world, talk of times past and things to come. What will become of this table when we move? There's certainly not space for it in the Carmichael Oaks apartment. And now I can't even start on the to-do list until I know the destiny of our memory-filled table.

I call my daughter, Sharon. "Do you want the dining room table?" I ask.

"Well … we could use the table. But don't Matt and Leesa want the table?"

"I don't know. They've got the big seminar table borrowed from Whitman College."

"But …"

"If you want it, I'd like to continue eating occasional holiday dinners on it."

"Doug's attached to the antique table."

"It's falling apart."

"I'll talk to him."

I should work through the stacks of immediate importance, but what I really want is to do something nice for the table. She's a little dry looking, with maybe a refried bean or two caked into a crack between the leaves, and a few light water spots from sweaty glasses. And there's that little scratch that caught my attention in the first place.

After a few half-hearted attempts at the list, I shove folders, lists, calendar, bills all to the right half of the table and rush, rush as if compelled, to the laundry room where I grab the Starbrite penetrating sealer-preserver teak oil and begin slathering it on the left half of the table. I take my time letting it soak in, then wipe off the excess as directed. Two more times of this regimen, then I cover the left side with a beach towel, move all the clutter from the right, and repeat the process. Much better. The water spots are gone. There's no trace left of the refried beans. A warm mellow glow emanates from freshly oiled teak. But ... there are still two small sections of the table, about the diameter of a Mason jar lid, that are dry looking. More oil. More elbow grease.

Finally, the table renewed, I turned my attention back to the list. The top item, circled in red, was "bank accounts."

According to the bankruptcy lawyer, I needed to walk away from the bank we'd used ever since moving to Gold River. The bank where we also had a loan account with a balance of over $10,000. The bank where they called me by name when I walked through the door. I was to set up a new account at a totally different bank.

It was time to stop procrastinating, to get on with things. I dialed the CalSTRS customer service number, canceled my automatic deposit and requested that my retirement check be delivered the old-fashioned way, by the U.S. postal service.

After I'd arranged to keep my CalSTRS check out of the banking system, I called back, relieved to get a different person on the other end of the phone. I identified myself as Michael Reynolds.

Although as a teenager I'd wished that my voice were more feminine sounding, over time I grew not only to accept it, but also to recognize that there were certain advantages to sometimes being heard as a "sir" on the phone. On that day, with CalSTRS, it was a definite advantage. I gave Mike's date of birth, his current address, and reeled off the now memorized last four digits of his Social Security number.

In less than half an hour I'd taken the beginning steps toward skipping out on scores of financial commitments—commitments made in all good faith. Less than half an hour to launch me down a path to becoming someone I never expected to be. I was stunned by the implications of what I'd just done. I felt shoddy.

A few years back in one of my many short-lived attempts at spiritual enlightenment, I attended a half-day meditation workshop. Now would be a good time to empty my mind, I thought. Though I hadn't practiced steadily enough to master the mind-emptying technique, it was worth a try. I straightened in my chair. Feet planted firmly on the floor, I took the requisite deep abdominal breaths, in, out, in, out. I let intruding thoughts pass through my too busy mind. My unfocused gaze rested on the table, newly aglow in the afternoon light. It was consoling. Maybe I, too, might someday be refurbished.

MOVING ON

May 2010

Walking back from dinner at the Richmonds', a path we'd walked under similar circumstances hundreds of times over the past decade, I was suddenly aware of the magnitude of the changes that were upon us. This would be the last night Mike and I would ever spend together in our Promontory Point home. I'd drive him to the SF airport around 1 the next morning (May 5), and when we backed out of the garage it would be the last time Mike would ever see the home that we'd so enjoyed for many years.

I'd arranged for Mike to spend the next 10 days with Jerry and Jackie, his brother and sister-in-law, in Tampa. The day before, while he was out with the Wards, I worked my way through all but the last three items on my to-do list:

- Pack Mike's clothes.
- Be sure he has I.D., cell phone, itinerary.
- Review directions to SF airport.
- Write note to be handed to ticket agent explaining that I need a "non-passenger escort pass."
- Put another note in an envelope for the flight attendants asking that they remind Mike not to get off the plane at the Denver stop.
- Come home from airport and pack house.
- Move to apartment before Mike's return.
- Don't look back.

On that walk home from the Richmonds' I reminded myself that although this last night was highly symbolic, the changes had already happened. We'd not really lived there, together, as partners, for the previous two years. The decisions were mine. The upkeep was mine. The financial responsibilities were mine. All of it was mine to balance, while Mike had the washing machine going endlessly, while Mike talked of wanting a Mercedes convertible, wanting to get his teeth straightened, let his hair grow to wear it in a ponytail, and go to Vienna, all while the wolf was at the door, and I was juggling. But on that soft spring night, walking the well-known path by the light of a more than half moon, Mike's warm hand in mine felt like the old Mike's hand, the familiar hand that had known and treated gently, every crease, every surface of my well-worn body. It would have been easier if that weren't the case.

The drive to the airport was traffic-free. I listened to a tribute to Howard Zinn on "City Arts & Lectures," a pleasant surprise that showed up on our local NPR station. Mike dozed.

At the check-in window I got a "non-passenger escort" I.D. and walked Mike to the gate where I could wait with him until he boarded the plane. I passed a prewritten note to a flight attendant asking that he remind Mike to stay on the plane during the Denver layover. Mike had no idea where or when to board, or how to get a boarding pass, or how to get from one terminal to the next, but he was willing to take direction. He would be fine. I hoped.

On my way home from the airport I stopped by the storage place and picked up the waiting boxes and tape, then drove home. I carried the boxes through the door that led from the garage, through the laundry room, to the kitchen. It was a little after 10. I hauled boxes into my office and started packing. I packed books from the built-in book shelves. I packed the framed covers that Mike had given to me after the publication of each book. Well, each book except for *Shut Up*, the 2009 publication that had escaped Mike's notice. I packed the "Save the Last Dance for Me" ceramic plaque with the image of a glamorous dancing couple, and the wooden sign that said "Well-Behaved Women Seldom Make History"—the first steps in the heartbreaking process of dismantling our decades together as full life partners

By noon friends had arrived with lunch and stayed on to pack. Carmichael Oaks provided five hours of Smooth Move services, and the owner of the company, Pam Landers, arrived in the early afternoon. Days before, when singer friends had taken Mike to lunch and a movie, Pam had come to the house to take pictures. A "certified relocation transition specialist," she'd walked through the house with me, measured furniture that I was hoping to take, then took snapshots of furniture, tables, picture placement and mirrors on walls, etc. Aware of Mike's condition, she knew that the more familiar the new place looked to him, the easier his transition would be. After she'd familiarized herself with our Promontory Point house, she and I went together to Carmichael Oaks. She measured rooms. We talked about possible furniture placement. She'd done 100 or so such moves during the past year, and no detail escaped her consideration. On that first packing day she brought more moving boxes, recycled from a previous move. She and a helper carefully removed and packed pictures and mirrors that were to go on the Carmichael Oaks walls, then took them over to the new place.

Piano movers arrived in the late afternoon and partially dismantled the piano, wrapping each section with heavy moving quilts, steadying the body of the instrument onto a dolly, and lifting it into the back of the truck where they securely strapped it to the side. Within the next hour or so, our piano was ensconced in the Carmichael Oaks living room style common area. It would remain our piano, but would live at Carmichael Oaks for as long as we did, or until we decided otherwise. I keep saying "we," but there was no more "we." Whatever the appropriate pronoun, the piano was moved and so, soon, would the rest of "us" be. My hope was that seeing his piano there would help with Mike's adjustment to the move.

There was now a big vacant space in the living room where the piano had stood, and boxes of china and crystal were packed, labeled, and sitting on the floor in front of the emptied bar cabinets.

Late in the afternoon, I got a call from Jerry in Tampa.

"We've got him home," Jerry told me. "I met him right when he got off the plane. We rode the tram to baggage claim. Jackie met us right there."

"Did he have his jacket and red carry-on?" I asked.

"He did. Beth and the girls are coming for dinner tonight. We'll do fine."

I relaxed, knowing that Mike was in good hands with his older brother.

With the help of friends, family, neighbors, box after box was packed and labeled. There were five destinations for boxes: Storage. Apartment. The Harveys' barn. Give Away. Consignment. Although I did some packing, I spent most of that time designating where each box was to go, and, too often, wandering aimlessly from one room to the next.

It would have been impossible to do any packing in Mike's presence. He would have held onto everything in sight. Over the years he had repeatedly said that he didn't want certain things ever to leave the family, or that he was never going to part with certain things, etc., etc. For the past several months I'd not even been able to put papers into the recycle bin without him dragging most of them back inside. Poor Mike. I suspected that his clinging ever more tightly to the things he could grasp physically meant that on an intuitive level he knew he was losing all that he'd been. He could no longer engage in meaningful conversation. He couldn't put two thoughts together. He couldn't drive. He couldn't direct singers. He couldn't make sense of times and locations in the newspaper movie listings. For him to be at the house during such chaos would have been excruciating. I was ever grateful to Jerry and Jackie for this 10-day break.

Sharon calls. They'll take the table. We'll gather around it on the coming Christmas Day, as will the spirits of so many others who've gathered around it over the decades. Altadena, Gold River, Woodacre. It doesn't matter. It will bring its essence with it wherever it goes.

May 2012

Dear Mike,

Yesterday evening, after Leesa and Mika went into the bedroom for their before-sleep reading time, Matt and I sat in their Walla Walla living room and talked about where and how to do your memorial. We didn't talk about when. When still seems a long way off, though we're both aware of a certain fragility that comes with the weight loss you've been experiencing.

We want to do justice to your whole life, your whole self, to remember so much more of you than now exists in your shell. I've arranged with UCSF for a brain autopsy. I believe that would have been your choice if we'd had this conversation 20 years ago. Such autopsies are so important for FTD research. Still, when it came time for me to sign on the dotted line, I could barely put pen to paper.

Sometimes it seems as if I'm watching this all from a distance, as if it's happening to some other couple. Not to us. Would that it were so. The "not to us" part. I would never wish this on any other couple in the world. Why am I even talking about wishes? The rain falls on everyone, and likewise shines the sun. Wishes have nothing to do with it. Hmmm. Did I just get Biblical?

Leesa graduates with a master's in social work next month. They've missed her work income for that past two-plus years, and they're now saddled with even more student loan debt, but I think they'll soon see some light at the end of the proverbial tunnel. Leesa already has a few part-time social work jobs. Now that she's graduated, there will be more coming her way. Matt and Leesa seem to have come through a stormy period with a new dedication to working things through. I'm relieved to see them being more affectionate and playful than I've seen in some time. You would be happy to see what good parents they both are.

Hoping to do right by you,
Marilyn

THE KINDEST LIE

May 2010

On the advice of "ours-for-life" Rachel, we worked on the kindest lie to tell Mike when he arrived at Carmichael Oaks after his Florida trip. In one of my many phone conversations with Mike, about halfway into his trip, I told him we'd received a notice from the homeowners association demanding that we repair our dry rot-infested fence or face a fine. Every day that I talked with Mike I added a few details. The fence guys found evidence of termites. The termite company found extensive infestation. The house needed to be tented. The next conversation would tell of evidence of toxic mold. I didn't know how much "stuck," but he did have some idea that not all was well with our house.

Our plan on Mike's return was that Matt would pick him up at the San Francisco airport. I would be at Carmichael Oaks waiting to greet them.

Although logic and reasoning was gone, Mike's intuitive side was more intact. One of his strengths had always been his capacity to connect with another's emotional distress. We hoped that if he thought I was in great emotional distress over the state of the house, he'd be his old, reassuring self. Here's the story Matt told when he met Mike at the airport:

He'd flown down to help me. He, Sharon, Doug, Cindi, Dale, Marg, etc., had to practically drag me out of the house. The house wasn't livable with all of the work they were doing on it. It was actually toxic. The only people who could go inside had to wear those haz-mat suits. But I was refusing to leave. He'd never seen me like that before. They'd had an emergency session with Dr. C and, with his help and the help of heavy-duty medication, they managed to get me settled into a nice residential hotel. They were lucky to find a place with a vacancy. Dr. C encouraged them to bring as much of our familiar furniture and things to the hotel as possible, so it would feel more like home to me. They got everything else into storage so it wouldn't be damaged by the chemicals and construction. I was doing a little better today. Matt thought I was really relieved that Mike was coming home, but he was worried about me. They had to do everything they could to reassure me. It would be months before the house would be livable again and I simply didn't seem to understand that.

WHEW!! During all of this someone asked, "What would happen if you just sat Mike down and explained to him what was happening, and that you had to move?"

I'm sure that would have been my question, too, if the tables had been turned. But after two-plus years of trying to explain things to Mike, and make sense of things, and talk through things, and do all of the things that once worked, I knew there was no way to deal truthfully with Mike in that situation.

The necessity of lies was, for me, one of the more difficult aspects of the whole mess. Although I enjoyed writing fiction, I'd always placed a high value on honesty in my real life. Now I found I was becoming more and more at ease lying to Mike. Would lying turn into a convenience that carried over to other aspects of my life? That was frightening to me.

The advice to tell the kindest lie was well taken, but looking back on that time I wonder: What were we thinking in conjuring that convoluted story? I suppose Rachel, or Felecia, the memory care director at Carmichael Oaks, had already told us at one point to keep things simple. The fewer details the better since the more details included the more confusing things become for someone with dementia. By that time, I'd already read numerous books about dementia—memoir, fiction, anything I could get my hands on. I'm pretty sure there was a unanimous opinion about keeping things simple. As much as I understood that in theory, it took a while for me to put the "keep it simple" tactic into practice. Even so, other than the effort it took for Matt to explain all of those details to Mike, there was no harm done. Matt's take on it was that Mike only listened to the first sentence anyway.

Matt tried to engage Mike in conversation on the drive back. How was Florida? Fine. Who did you see while you were there? Everyone. How's Uncle Jerry doing? Fine. Mike soon went to sleep and stayed asleep until they pulled up in front of Carmichael Oaks. I'd been watching for them from the "living room" and rushed out to greet Mike as he got out of the car. He gave me a quick hug, then stood under the portico, taking in the entrance to the facility. Looking confused and worried he asked, "Do we live here now?"

"Just for a while," I said.

Matt got Mike's bag from the car and the three of us took the elevator to the third floor. Inside the apartment I pointed to his treasured paintings, showed him the bedroom, complete with all of the bedroom furniture from Promontory Point. The closet space, the two bathrooms, the balcony with two chairs, plants, and a fountain. When I asked if he didn't think we could live here for a little while, he nodded, said he was tired, and went to bed.

We couldn't believe how easy that had been! All of our fretting, and worrying, and story conjuring! Matt and I were not the only ones who'd been so concerned. Dale and Marg were eager to hear how things went, as were Sharon and Doug, Cindi, Jeannie and Bill, and a host of others. After Matt and I sharing our relief to the point of near-giddiness, he went back to Dale and Marg's where he was staying. From there he sent a group email, reporting the easy re-entry. The next morning Dale, Marg, Matt, and Sharon met us for breakfast downstairs in the dining room. In terms of Mike's responses to family and close friends, it still remained the more the merrier, and we wanted to keep Mike as merrier as possible.

Of course, I knew this easy entry might have been the calm before the storm, but I was quite happy with the calm, however long it might last.

GOODBYE, GOLD RIVER

May 2010

Two nights before Mike's return from Florida, I spent the night at Carmichael Oaks. There was still much to be done at the house, but the C.O. apartment was put together. Two accent walls were painted, the one in the living room was a "burnt caramel," in the bedroom "sage green." All of the boxes that contained things to be moved to the apartment had been unpacked and recycled. Pictures and mirrors were in place, fresh flowers were on the table that divided the kitchen from the living room. Clothes were hanging in the closets, towels and sheets in the little linen cabinet. The bed was made. It did all have a familiar look. Anyone who had been in our house more than once or twice could have come in here and thought, "Mike and Marilyn live here."

Two chairs, a little table, and a few plants were on the balcony just outside the living room sliders. The balcony overlooked a broad driveway that divided Carmichael Oaks from a large acute care facility. It wasn't a pretty view, but if one looked in the right direction, from the right angle, there were oak trees and sky to be seen.

Mike's desk fit easily opposite our bed, as did the small rolling file cabinet from my downstairs office. All but the most current and immediately necessary files would go to storage. That hadn't been done yet.

A little before 10, I took Sunny for a walk through the courtyard and down to a grassy area outside the assisted living section. She sniffed around with great interest—nothing like new scents to fascinate a dog. She found the spot that would become her toilet. I cleaned up after her and dropped her package in a nearby container. Back at the apartment we settled in for the night, she in her familiar bed beside the desk, and I in my familiar bed on the opposite side of the room.

I slept surprisingly well that first night. It probably helped that I'd been working nonstop from early in the morning until late at night since the morning I'd seen Mike off to Florida. I woke early, walked Sunny, and tried out the shower in what would become "my" bathroom. There were two bathrooms in this apartment, a luxury neither of the more upscale places we visited could offer.

Breakfast at 7. I was greeted cheerfully by Ronnie who asked my name, told me of breakfast options (plenty) and took my order. I had grapefruit, one poached egg, bacon, toast and coffee. It was all good. Halfway through breakfast Janice came into the dining room, greeting people by name. She brought a cup of coffee to my table, asked how things were going and if there was anything I needed. The dining room quickly filled up. There was lots of chatter. Most of the people looked to be 10 to 20 years older than I. That was okay. I've always liked old people.

After breakfast I went back to the house and continued packing. No one room was completely empty yet. The guest room was totally intact. Matt and Leesa would be taking the queen-sized bed and the linens and pillows that went with it. The chest that was Sharon and Doug's to begin with would go back to them. The clothes it contained— extra bathing suits for the grandkids from years past, assorted winter things, extra pajamas—all could go to Goodwill. I boxed it up and labeled it.

Friends arrived to pack more dishes and crystal. Those boxes would go to the barn. In the afternoon Felicia, a local musician friend with whom Mike had happily worked for many years, dropped by with her adult son, Barry. When she'd told me that Barry had sold rocks from his garden on Craigslist, I asked if I could hire him to sell some of my things. I didn't know the first thing about maneuvering such sales, but I had a number of things that I thought might be sold in that way. Felicia arranged for Barry to come over the next day to check things out.

As we went from room to room, Barry jotted down notes and I identified what I wanted to sell. I'd already talked with each of the kids about what they wanted. The wrought iron and glass coffee table plus patio furniture to Cindi. The guest room bed, martini couch, Mike's black leather chair, washer dryer and assorted smaller pieces to Matt and Leesa. A few decorative items and the dining room set to Sharon and Doug. Occasional chairs, bar stools, side tables, a few lamps, more patio furniture, vases, pots, a file cabinet, a rice cooker, large pots and pans that I expected never to use again, a coffeemaker with bells and whistles, footstools, a printer, hoses, garden tools, so much of our lives—all to Craigslist.

Barry arranged a time to come back with his van. He took everything to his place and sold it from there. I offered him a 50/50 cut. He said he didn't want anything. We haggled. I was so overwhelmed with the moving process and all that went with it, I knew that left to my own devices I'd probably end up giving it all away. Anything he brought in was more than I'd have had without his help. We agreed to disagree for a while and work things out later. He loaded his van.

That night, before Sunny and I went back to the apartment, I took a nearly full bottle of Chardonnay and a blue plastic cup upstairs to our almost empty bedroom. The little portable stereo was still there, sitting on the floor, as were a few CDs. I got cushions from the sofa bed in the bedroom we'd called Mike's office and piled them on the floor. I opened the shutters on the window that looked out over Promontory Point. I started Emmylou Harris's "Stumble Into Grace" album, poured wine into the cup, sat on the cushions and stared out the window at the familiar scene. The tops of redwood trees, the moon bright and full—a clear, crisp night, like so many other clear, crisp nights had been. One of the things we'd both loved about this upstairs bedroom was that even with the windows wide open and uncovered, we were in a private space, breathing in the scent of pine that filtered in through the open windows.

I refilled the plastic cup and scooted down so I was resting my back against the cushions. I let my mind wander to happier times in this room, the window open, a mild breeze freshening the air, us curled together under a light sheet, laughing maybe. Loving maybe. Loss washed through me, hollowed my inner being. The plaintive voice of Emmylou sang that even though her lover was standing on the other side of the river, he could still see her face. She will be standing there forever. The verse ends with the plaintive question, "Why won't you look at me? Here I am. Here I am."

We'd bought this album shortly after it was released, back when Mike was fully Mike. For a while it had been one of our go-to albums when we were in the car. At the time we simply enjoyed the music and appreciated the poetry of the lyrics. Now, though, I was struck by how strongly I identified with the person who was standing by the river, her love on the other side. Why wouldn't he look at her?

It seemed Mike had been on the other side of the river for such a long, long time. It'd been such a long, long time since he'd looked at me, since he'd truly seen my face, since he'd heard my plea. I lay there sobbing, catching my breath and sobbing. I turned my face into the cushions and surrendered to the force of grief. I felt Sunny inching close to me, until she was lying next to my stretched out legs, her head resting against my thigh.

The Mike with whom I bought "Stumble Into Grace," with whom I listened to it in the car, the Mike who did once see me, and hear me, and love me, was gone. I knew that. I'd known that for a long time, but maybe the certainty of that knowledge came in stages—at first knowing, but not believing. Then knowing, but still hoping. Then knowing, but not feeling. Finally, knowing, believing, feeling, hopeless.

I reached for Sunny and rubbed behind her ears. She scooted closer. The wine. Emmylou. I knew I was becoming maudlin. I didn't give a shit. I'd not cried, really full-out cried, for months. I poured the rest of the wine and let the next song wash over me, the one that imagines her love as her "dear companion." Imagines that "I'm the one you cling to/And your voice still calls my name …"

I cried over that, too.

Sunny still at my side, I lay propped against the cushions, half-listening to the rest of the album, half-seeing what was beyond the window, half-wondering what would become of us.

After a while in silence, I rose and walked to the double sinks and vanity that formed the short leg of an L off what was our bedroom. Only what we would need in the apartment had been taken from these cabinets. I grabbed an empty box and pulled out a wide variety of unopened travel shampoos, conditioners, lotions. I added an unopened package of four rolls of toilet paper and several plastic bags collected from trips to the dentist. Those all contained one toothbrush, one container of floss, and one small tube of toothpaste. All but one of those bags went into the packing box. I took a new toothbrush and tube of toothpaste from the remaining bag and brushed the aftertaste of wine from my mouth. I taped the box closed, labeled it "Loaves and Fishes," then, with Sunny following close behind, I carried the box, and the plastic cup, and empty wine bottle downstairs.

It was over. So much was over.

November 21, 2014

Dear Mike,

The mornings are cold now, 51 degrees when I got up—not cold to someone in Rochester, NY, I'm sure, but to an old Southern California girl, it feels like Siberia. These days I'm more cold-blooded than ever. This morning I woke up around 6 and lay in bed, clothed in my makeshift pajamas, jersey workout pants, a long-sleeved turtleneck shirt under a short-sleeved T-shirt, heavy socks and fingerless gloves, under the bedspread comforter and both of Aunt Ruth's quilts. You would laugh, if you could.

I lay there all warm and toasty, dreading getting up to the cold, remembering how you were always the first one out of bed, getting the house warmed up, starting the coffee. Remembering how, when I was pregnant with Matt, you would go out and start my car five minutes before leaving time, so it would be warm by the time I left for Wilson High School.

How happy you were with that pregnancy. I was barely three weeks late and yes, because I was regular as clockwork, it was likely I was pregnant. We had, after all, been "trying" for two months.

"We're going to have a baby!" you'd said, beaming.

"Maybe, but let's not say anything until we know for sure."

You just stood there, smiling.

My first pregnancy, with the other guy, had ended in a miscarriage—a spontaneous abortion was the official term. It was propitious. I was pregnant again, six months later, and it was Baby Sharon who came down the chute. There would be no Sharon if the first pregnancy had lasted. It makes me sad just to think of a Sharon-less world.

You knew the first pregnancy story, and I reminded you that the first trimester could be iffy.

"We shouldn't tell anyone until after three months. Okay?"

"Okay," you said.

It was a Sunday and we were having dinner with my mother. We walked into a house smelling of pot roast. Lace doilies on the backs and arms of every piece of upholstered furniture. With only one foot through the door, before even saying hello, you called to my mother, "Marilyn's pregnant!"

My mother got teary-eyed; the girls jumped around, hugging me.

"When are you due?" my mother asked.

"In about 10 months," I told her, but the cat was out of the bag, and there was no putting it back. And I was indeed pregnant, and we got Baby Matt.

With Sharon and Cindi aged 10 and 9, I'd not been eager to add another child into the mix. The girls were at good ages, easy to care for and fun. As much as I enjoyed those earlier stages, life was easier with them half-grown. Being the quintessential late bloomer, at 33 I was in my first year of teaching, not eager to interrupt that hard-won career start. Fair was fair, though—nothing you ever tossed up to me, but what I knew in my heart. You'd generously and willingly taken on the father role, officially adopting Sharon and Cindi shortly after we married. I owed you a baby. And then there was Matt, the gift that goes on giving.

But I was talking about the morning temperature, wasn't I? I was thinking about the small comforts that I sometimes miss. The warming of the house while I'm still in bed. The coffee ready for me when I stumble into the kitchen. The gentle laughter at eccentricities such as my sleeping attire.

Last week when I was in Walla Walla, I walked to town—all sorts of bright-leafed trees showing off in the yards of old fashioned homes. My first stop was that delightful little independent bookstore, the one you walked out of when my back was turned and we didn't find you for over an hour. That was our last visit there together. But I'm talking about a recent trip, when no one got lost.

I must have been in there for over an hour, browsing literary fiction, the YA section (no Marilyn Reynolds books there), biographies and memoir. I felt guilty not buying, knowing that I'd gone to the dark side of ebooks on my iPad. I will be sad when that corner becomes vacant, as it surely will within the next decade or two, but, as with the greater selection/lower priced supermarkets that drove small, independent stores out of business in the '50s, including Daddy's market, such progress seems inevitable.

I did buy something, though. Unlike Ann Patchett's bookstore in Tennessee that is only a bookstore, the front part of the Walla Walla store has turned into something like a variety five and dime, only higher priced, with toys and calendars, greeting cards and gadgets. I bought a "bear claw" backscratcher for $7. It has a shiny chrome, five-pronged claw-like top with a telescoping handle that allows for an extension of from one to three feet. It's to manage that lost small comfort of your back scratching talents.

It's only been within the last two years that I've been able to spend $7 on an unnecessary item without breaking into a sweat. The one silver lining to paying nearly

$40,000 a year for your care is that all of our withheld income tax dollars come back in refunds—an enforced savings that provides a cushion for inevitable car repair bills and the occasional trip to Southern California or Walla Walla. Last summer I joined the rest of the family on vacation at a resort in Oregon—not cheap, but as the American Express ads say, priceless. For over 20 years I had one of those no limit American Express cards. No more. No more credit cards at all. I like that, though I know it's a good idea to have at least one card for emergencies.

On my last Alaska Airlines trip I filled out a form for a Visa card. They were offering thousands of bonus miles plus a free round trip to anywhere in the world that they and their partner airlines fly. I expect to get the rejection in the mail any day now. It seems bankruptcy doesn't look good on the credit reports.

Ramble, ramble. It's as if I were truly talking with you, relaxed in front of the fireplace, or on one of those long drives between here and Woodacre. That's another of the small comforts I'm missing—someone to take pleasure in my rambles. Someone to fasten the clasp on my necklace, zip up the back of my dress, check the bump on my butt that I can't see for myself, pick me up when I take my car in for repair, change the audio book CDs when I'm driving or drive while I manage maps and CDs.

It's time to put up Christmas lights, get a tree, drag out the wreaths and the choristers, the photo albums of Christmases past, all of those things you did with such great enthusiasm. Or to be more accurate, overdid with great enthusiasm. As you once could have predicted, without you my decorations will be minimal and there will be no special color scheme. I didn't keep all the ornaments from the purple Christmas, or the gold Christmas, or the silver Christmas, and I won't be buying new garlands and fresh wreaths. But even though my minimalist approach suits me, I miss your enthusiasm. The place would be decorated by now, though I can't really imagine you in this new place. This new life. I can only still imagine you scratching my back, or picking me up from the car repair place, or fastening the clasp on a necklace. Really, though, I don't wear necklaces anymore anyway.

It's getting harder to write to you. The you I write to, the old you, is becoming more and more distant—our lives together slipping further away with each passing day. I will always appreciate those times and who you were, but dwelling in those times doesn't fit with the necessary reinvention of myself. You will show up when the Christmas lights come out of the box tangled in such a way that it would be easier for two to untangle, or when I can't reach the top of the tree to place the gaudy star up there. I did keep that gaudy star. And you'll show up tomorrow morning, when the house is cold and the coffee's not ready. You'll never be forgotten. You'll continue to show up often. But, forgive me, you don't get to stay long.

Marilyn

IT'S NOT TIME!

May 2010

Because Sunny no longer has easy access to an outdoor area at Carmichael Oaks, she and I soon develop a habit of early morning walks. There's still a lot that needs to be cleared out of the house and, since Mike generally sleeps until 8 or after these days, my pattern is to walk Sunny around 6 or 6:30 in the morning, then take her with me to Promontory Point for an hour or so of packing and organizing while Mike still sleeps. But on this particular morning we've only been at the house for a few minutes when I get a call from the front desk person saying that Mike has been standing out front waiting for someone. Maybe he's confused about the time?

"Is he wearing a tuxedo?"

"Yes."

"Would you please ask him to come to the phone so I can talk with him?"

When Mike picks up, he says he's been waiting for Don, who usually picks him up for Camerata rehearsals, but Don never came.

"The concert isn't until tomorrow," I tell him.

"I don't know where Don is," he says in that angry voice that is now nearly standard.

"It isn't time. Just go back upstairs. I'll be there in a few minutes."

"Okay. I'll just wait here."

"No. Go on back to the apartment. I'll be there soon."

"Okay. I'll wait here."

I lift Sunny into the car and rush back to Carmichael Oaks. Mike is standing out front, in his tuxedo, with his music folder, waiting. He gets in the car, and I drive the half-block or so to our designated parking spot.

"Aren't you going to take me to the concert?"

"It's not until tomorrow."

"Oh, okay," he says, not sounding convinced.

Knowing that Mike no longer understands time, and knowing that he's anxious not to be late to whatever is coming up—a rehearsal, dinner, any appointment—I struggle to be patient, to tamp down my irritation.

Back at the apartment I suggest he put on other, more comfortable clothes, which he does, reluctantly. Eight in the morning is a little early to do the sort of shopping I have planned for the day—a few more over-the-door hooks from Organize It, some things from Trader Joe's for when Jeannie and Bill will join us early in the evening for drinks and appetizers. But errands seem the best defense against Mike's desire to be picked up in his tuxedo 30 hours ahead of time. We go to the market for a red bell pepper. We drop a few things off at the cleaners. We drive to Organize It. Not open until 10. We go to Target—open at 9—to replace our topless martini shaker. On to Best Buy, where I want to look at small desktop printers. Not open until 10. We drive, very slowly, to O'Brot Café in Folsom, where we sip lattes and I count the minutes until the outlet stores will open. Once the little hand is on 10 and the big hand on 12, we enter the Bose outlet where we (I) find and purchase a much-needed upgrade to our ancient portable boom box. Back to Organize It, then to Carmichael Oaks and our apartment, where Mike immediately dons his tuxedo and wants me to take him to the concert.

"Not yet," I tell him.

"I'm going!"

"It's not time."

He takes his jacket off, throws it on the floor, and stomps into the bedroom. I call out after him, "Grow up!" Not helpful, I know. After a few minutes I suggest that Mike dress more casually for lunch. He puts on shorts and a short-sleeved shirt. We go downstairs to lunch, come back, and Mike puts on his tuxedo.

To quote Kurt Vonnegut, so it goes.

DAILY LIFE AT CARMICHAEL OAKS

June 2010

A month into our stay at Carmichael Oaks, all of the dining room waitstaff knew us by name, and knew what we were likely to order. As seems to be the custom in these places, we soon learned to sit at the same table for every meal.

At the giant aquarium places, residents in independent living have their own separate dining room, away from the walkers and wheelchairs of those in assisted living. Here at our 6-foot-by-5-foot aquarium place, the only separate dining area was in memory care, a "secure" section. There were times when Mike would watch an aide wheel someone in from assisted living, push him or her—usually her—up close to the table, secure a bib, then, when food arrived, feed her, small spoonful by small spoonful. He would scan the room, focusing particularly on the most frail of the diners, then loudly announce, "I don't want to stay in this convalescent home!" Other times he would be oblivious to all but the food on the plate in front of him.

There were fresh linen tablecloths every day in the giant aquarium places. Here at C.O., the white linen tablecloths were protected by clear glass table tops and changed once a week. The only problem with that was that residents some-times found it convenient to wipe their hands on the unprotected segment of tablecloth that hung near their laps. But this was a minor flea bite of a problem compared to the now simmering-just-below-a-boil water in the soup pot.

On this particular morning, our favorite waiter, Ernesto, has recommended the blueberry pancakes to us. I'm more of a poached-egg-on-toast person, but Mike loves pancakes and Ernesto learned that early on. Mike soaks the pan-cakes with syrup, slathers them with whipped cream, finishes them off in a flash, and stands to leave.

Back in No. 324, I get him set up with a movie on the classics channel. I tell him I have to drop some materials off to Kathy—someone he knows I've been working with, or at least did know that a while back. I tell him I'll be back by 11.

In reality I'm wanting to get a much-needed hour or so of work done back at the house, but the less said to Mike about the house the better.

About 15 minutes into packing leftover items from the guest room, Mike calls. "I don't know where you are!"

"I'm taking some things to Kathy. I should be back by 11."

"Well, okay. I just don't know what's happening."

I repeat what I've just said, trying to be as reassuring as possible. Ten minutes later there's another phone call—same thing. I talk with Mike four times in less than an hour, each time a near verbatim copy of the time before. I'm upstairs gathering things for the Goodwill when Mike's fifth phone call comes in. I don't rush to pick up the phone, knowing I'll be back at the apartment within a few minutes anyway.

In the car I listen to Mike's message from his unanswered call.

"Marilyn. I don't know where you are! WHERE THE FUCK ARE YOU?"

I call back. "I just picked up your message. You don't get to talk to me like that."

"Okay! OKAY!! FORGET IT!"

On my way back, a few blocks from Carmichael Oaks, there's Mike, walking/stomping along busy Fair Oaks Boulevard at a rapid pace, Sunny, unleashed, following close behind. I make a U-turn, pull to the side of the road, get out, call to Sunny and get her in the car, then open the door wide on the passenger side. Mike gets in and slams the door with all his might. He jerks at the seatbelt, which makes it impossible to secure. He repeats that motion several times before he finally slows down enough to actually get the belt fastened.

"Where were you going?"

"Home! I'm going home!"

"We can't do that yet."

"I want a divorce!"

"Okay," I tell him, allowing myself a moment in which to fantasize about a longed-for freedom.

When we return to the apartment, we each hover in our separate corners. Around noon I suggest that Mike go downstairs for a bite to eat.

"No, I'll wait for you," he says.

"We're getting a divorce," I tell him. "I won't be sharing meals with you."

He waits around for a few minutes, then goes downstairs to the dining room. I pretty much lay low until the sing-along, where Mike exudes warmth, and charm.

I wish I only had to see him in public.

NOT QUITE KEEPING
TRACK OF MIKE

July through December 2010

By July, we were in something of a routine at Carmichael Oaks—breakfast at 7:30, lunch at noon, dinner at 5. We didn't have to eat at those times. The dining room was open for a span of three hours for each meal. But Mike had fallen into a pattern, and any deviation from a pattern was troublesome to him.

The details of everyday life were definitely easier at C.O. The freedom from providing three meals a day for us was welcome. It meant fewer trips to the grocery store, where Mike would sometimes grab strange items to deposit in our shopping cart. Or worse yet, where he would wander away. The small kitchen with just a refrigerator and microwave was infinitely more manageable than the fully stocked Gold River kitchen with countertop stove, oven, and a myriad of small appliances on the center island, available for whatever task Mike might conjure. If there were times when the C.O. dining room food bordered on boring, it was worth a bit of boredom not to have to be on the three-meals-a-day job, or to be monitoring Mike's kitchen activities. And really, as far as the food went, their cooks were at least as good as I was, often better.

No longer able to leave Mike on his own long enough to participate in my local writing group, I started a new group at C.O. We met once a week in the "library," which was directly across from our apartment. I'd get Mike set up with a movie, then walk across the hall to meet with fellow writers. Sooner or later, usually sooner, Mike would come looking for me. As soon as our apartment door opened, I could call to him. He might come in and sit with us for a moment, or go on downstairs to the area where doughnuts were always available. Better still, he might go to the downstairs living room and play the piano for a while. He was always restless, but his level of anxiety was lower when I was on the premises than if I were elsewhere.

There were six of us in the writing group. I was the youngest at 74. The others ranged in age from 85 to 96. Each meeting, I brought in a writing prompt, which they (me, too) would respond to during the week. We'd bring what we'd written to the next meeting. Each person read his/her work to the group, and we responded to what we liked in the reading. The 96-year-old had severe vision problems. She wrote with the help of various magnifying devices, then, because the actual writing too small to read, I read her work aloud for her.

The writers regularly expressed their appreciation for our group. To a person each said it was the highlight of his/her week. Truly, though, the group was a gift to me—moments of sanity in the midst of disorder and instability.

Although Mike and I left Carmichael Oaks in January 2011, I continued meeting with the C.O. writing group on a biweekly basis for five more years. Ica Ingraham, the oldest member of the group, died in November 2015 at the age of 102. Her niece now has volumes of Ica's tales of her life growing up on a farm in Iowa, hilarious stories of camping mishaps with her husband and friends, and stories of sweet and tender times. All of the writers were aging courageously, and I was lucky to know them on a deeper level than the hellos and goodbyes in the dining room setting.

One of the noticeable changes in Mike's behaviors was that he visited the bathroom much more frequently than in previous years, and he rushed in with apparent great urgency. In the car he would ask that I stop so he could pee. If there wasn't a filling station immediately available, he would demand that I let him out so he could pee at the side of the road. Surface street. Freeway. It didn't matter. He demanded that I stop the car "right now!" to let him out. Thank the Goddess for child safety locks on car doors. There was no apparent physical reason for this increased frequency. He didn't have a urinary tract infection or other urological problems. It was likely related to FTD, and perhaps a precursor to incontinence.

In September we flew to Walla Walla to visit Matt, Leesa and Mika. Mike was up and down several times on the flight to Seattle, going back to the restrooms, then immediately returning to his seat. "There was a line," he said at one point. Then he was up again. And back again.

As we began our descent into Seattle, Mike unbuckled his seat belt and said he had to use the restroom. The seat belt light was on. Everyone was to stay seated.

"You can't go now," I told him.

"I have to," he said and walked toward the back of the plane.

The attendant sent him back to his seat and again announced the necessity of everyone remaining in their seats with safety belts buckled until we'd landed and the captain turned off the seat belt sign.

Then Mike got up and walked toward the front of the plane. He was sent back. There was another announcement. When he again unbuckled his seat belt, I held his arm and told him he really must stay in his seat. I watched as he put his carry-on bag on his lap, then seemed to relax. I realized he'd peed in his pants.

Once off the plane, I asked Mike if he wanted to use the restroom. No, he said, he'd already done that.

"Which way to baggage claim?" he asked.

"We won't get our bags until we get to Walla Walla. Seattle is just a stop-over…. Are you hungry?"

The answer to that was always yes, and food was always a successful, even if short-lived, distraction. We got a small pizza and sat down to eat. After just a few bites Mike got up, said he'd be right back and rushed away. I thought he'd gone to the restroom, but when he wasn't back after 10 minutes, I became concerned. I got our stuff—his jacket and carry-on, my briefcase with computer, purse and jacket, and went to the gate from which we were to depart. He wasn't there. I went to customer service and explained the problem. They paged Mike, but asking him to return to gate C2D was as effective as leaving him a message in Swahili would have been. I provided his description and went looking for him. At this point I longed for the bright red wool jacket he'd worn all last winter. On this day he was wearing what 99 percent of the other middle-aged men in the airport were wearing—dark long-sleeved shirt and dark pants. I called Mike's cell phone, which I'd watched him put in his pocket when we left the apartment. I got his voice mail.

Somewhere along the way it occurred to me that he had probably been uncomfortable in his wet pants and gone looking for his suitcase. I went to airport security with this idea. They advised contacting Seattle Port Police and reporting him missing. They made the call for me. Two police officers arrived within minutes. They were thorough and reassuring, took my cell phone number and went on the search.

As I'd guessed, he'd gone looking for our bags. The police found him outside the security area. One of the officers escorted Mike back to the gate where I was waiting. He was carrying someone else's suitcase.

"I didn't know where you were!" he shouted.

I thanked the officer profusely, then told him the bag Mike was carrying was not his.

"Here, I'll put this back where it belongs," he said, motioning toward the suitcase. Mike handed it to him and we walked through the gate, the last two to board the plane to Walla Walla.

Later in the week we visited a local bookstore. Mike was looking at "coffee table" books and I was looking for a birthday card for a friend. When I was ready to pay for the card, I looked around the store and Mike wasn't there. I set the card down and went out to the sidewalk, scanning the area in both directions. No sign of Mike. Back in the bookstore I asked if any of the clerks had noticed him leave. He was wearing a red sweatshirt, I told them. Nope. One of the clerks had noticed him in the store but hadn't seen him leave.

I left the store and headed back the way we'd come, looking in all the little shops of the sort that appealed to Mike. I called both Matt and Leesa at work. Leesa took an early lunch to join the search. My hope was that Mike had gone back to their house, about a 20-minute walk from downtown. But when I got there, he still was not to be found. Leesa also had no luck in finding him. I kept calling Mike's cell phone but, although he often carried it, he seldom turned it on or checked messages anymore.

About half an hour—seemingly days—after I got back to Matt and Leesa's, Mike came walking through the door.

"Where were you?" he demanded.

"Looking for you until I didn't know where else to look. We were about to call the police."

"I didn't know where to find you!" he shouted.

The flights home were uneventful—"uneventful" being the new definition of paradise. In fact, the trip back was *so* uneventful that I felt emboldened to try another flight with Mike, this time to Los Angeles. I'd been invited to participate in the September "celebration" of banned books at the Santa Monica library.

Nancy Obrien, our longtime singer/traveler friend, met up with us near the library. The three of us had breakfast at the Tudor Tea Shoppe in honor of English breakfasts shared years ago on our walk through the Cotswolds. As was prearranged, I left Mike in Nancy's care so I could check in at the library and take my place among other writers of banned books.

After a walk with her dogs and a visit to a mall, Nancy brought Mike to the library just in time for my talk about being the author of Young Adult books that are sometimes banned. Other friends had also dropped by to cheer me on. The event was held outside under a temporary canopy and consisted mainly of readings of banned materials, some by the authors and some by others reading works of those no longer around to read for themselves, Mark Twain, Jack London, and J.D. Salinger among them.

It was a sparkling Southern California day, the sky such a bright blue, the clouds such a pure white, it was difficult to imagine that air quality could ever be a concern. Mike was attentive, laughing in all the right places, and, later, over lunch at a little outdoor beachfront cafe, he participated in the conversation, asking about our friends' families, commenting on the food, seemingly as right as ever. I was surprised and relieved that things went so smoothly.

The plane to take us from Burbank to Sacramento was delayed by over an hour. Mike's anxiety level rose by the minute during our long wait. He wanted to stand in line for whatever plane was boarding in the general vicinity of our gate and was mistrustful of my assurance that the plane to Portland, or wherever, was not our plane. The wait that was just an hour in real time soon felt like somewhere between six months and eternity.

Finally, landing in Sacramento, Mike grabbed the first suitcase from the baggage carousel and proceeded out the door with it.

"Mike," I called, running after him. He stopped and looked at me.

"That's not our suitcase," I said, taking his arm and guiding him back to the baggage carousel. He didn't resist when took the suitcase from him, but in the time it took for me to place it back on the carousel, he'd grabbed another one and was headed for the door. I brought him, and it, back. He took another and another wrong suitcase from the belt. I put another and another back.

It was so tedious, this life I was now living. I had to be constantly alert, trying to avoid potential trouble, ready to do damage control. I was tired, and there was no end in sight. On the other hand, we'd made the trip without any major problems, and it was great reconnecting with longtime friends, and being an author out in the world again.

Based on Dr. Hess's recommendation, Mike had recently stopped taking Aricept and had the dosage of Ritalin lowered by half. As far as we could tell, the Aricept had not been staving off any cognitive decline. The stimulant, Ritalin, had been prescribed some time back when ADD was still being considered as a possible cause of some of Mike's mix-ups. Although Ritalin was not indicated for dementia, Mike did seem less apathetic when he was taking it. With the change in meds, he had become slightly more engaged, often asking to go "home." He also resumed his habit of six months or so earlier, reading reports of the weather in Vienna and Paris, in preparation for "coming travels." None of this was a problem. It was just indicative of the puzzling shifts in Mike's thought processes.

One of FTD's many possible symptoms is an extreme hunger for sweets, a symptom that Mike was exhibiting. He had been wolfing down the always available doughnuts from the lobby, or cookies from the snack bar, or ice cream if he could find it. Mike had always had a sweet tooth, especially for pie or pastries, but he'd never been prone to overindulging. Now "overindulging" was an understatement.

In the slippage department, I heard from three different residents that they saw Mike trying to get into the apartment directly below us. This happened when he returned from singing in the memory care section of our complex. Luckily, that apartment was vacant, so there was no harm done. This mix-up was partly my fault.

Mike had done well using the elevator to get to our floor and finding his way back to our apartment from the dining room, or memory care, or his piano in the downstairs living room. But because he'd put on so much weight and was getting so little exercise, I got us started using the stairs instead of the elevator. That, of course, worked fine when I was with him. But it turned out that coming back from memory care on his own, Mike had been stopping at the second floor rather than taking the next set of stairs up to the third floor. On the second floor, he'd go to the apartment directly below us and try to get in.

When a new resident moved in below us, Mike's attempts to get into her apartment frightened her. Once, when she opened the door a crack to see who was there, Mike pushed his way past her and demanded to know where his dog was. Another time he made his way in through the sliders that opened onto her balcony.

Although I knew Mike's doughnut eating wasn't a healthy practice, going downstairs to the doughnut counter was something he could manage on his own. I was grateful for *anything* he could manage on his own and I expect it was, on some level of awareness, a relief to him to have 10 minutes free from my watching his every move. But even that tiny piece of autonomy came into question when he came back from a doughnut run, keys in hand, very irritated, and said to me, "I couldn't get in!"

"Get in where?"

"Here! I couldn't get in!"

"Well … I was here. The door wasn't locked."

"I'm telling you I couldn't get in!!!"

Then, clothes on, including shoes, he got into bed.

Common wisdom holds that it's best to hear the emotion rather than the words. I too often got stuck on the words. I should simply have said something like, "Let's get your key checked," or "How's the doughnut?"

Moments after Mike went to bed, the phone rang. It was one of the staff saying that Mike had been trying to get into the apartment below us. When his key wouldn't work, he gave the door a hard kick, once again frightening the little lady who lived there.

"We really can't have this," she told me.

"I know," I said. It was more and more obvious that neither I nor the C. O. staff could sufficiently monitor Mike's behavior.

No matter how hard I tried, I couldn't always keep track of Mike. I took showers. I went to the bathroom. I put clothes in the washer down the hall from us. These things all offered opportunities for Mike to get away, to rush out on the busy street, or force his way into another apartment, or do any number of unpredictable, dangerous things.

The thought of moving Mike to a "secure" facility, a place where he would live behind locked doors and gates, was horrifying. On the other hand, it was clear that the day would come when we would be asked to leave the Carmichael Oaks facility. I didn't even want to think about it, but I had to start carefully considering alternatives. And honestly, as much as I hated the thought of what was ahead for Mike, I knew it would be a great relief for me not to be watching out for him, micromanaging him, day in and day out.

PASQUALE'S ON FOOT

September 2010

It was not long after our trip to Santa Monica that Mike disappeared from Carmichael Oaks. He was watching TV when I left around 3 to meet a friend for coffee. I told him I wouldn't be gone long and reminded him that we had plans to meet friends at 6 for dinner at a little Italian place about a mile down the road.

He barely looked up as I left. I thought I could get away with a 45-minute absence. Engrossed in conversation, I didn't check my watch until it was nearly 4:30. I should have set an alarm. I hurried back to the apartment. Mike wasn't there. I went downstairs, hoping to find him playing the piano. Not there. I checked the dining room. None of the servers had seen him since lunchtime. No one at the front desk knew where he was. The director, Janice, called the downstairs caregivers and asked that they search the building, including storage areas and laundry rooms.

Mike still sometimes asked to go "home," but was usually easily redirected from that idea. But there was that time he'd taken off walking, headed for "home."

Maybe … I stopped by the front office on my way out, telling Janice I was going to check at the old house. I asked her to call my cell phone if she learned anything new.

Now dusk, I drove along busy Fair Oaks Boulevard, scanning for Mike on both sides of the street. I pulled into the garage of our old, empty house. The key was still in its hiding place and I doubted that, if Mike had used it, he would have put it back. Nothing, though, was predictable. I went inside, calling for Mike. There was a light on, but I was pretty sure I'd left it on from the last time I'd been there, clearing out our remaining belongings for storage.

I looked in every room upstairs and down, but there was no sign of Mike. In the car, on my way back to Carmichael Oaks, I called the director to say I'd had no luck. She said the activities director had seen Mike go out front some time between 3:30 and 4, but thought nothing of it since he often would get picked up out front for rehearsals, or movies or lunch with friends.

Even before FTD, Mike was not a careful pedestrian. Now it was dark, and I imagined the worst. In the midst of giving Janice a description of what Mike had been wearing so she could pass that on when she called the police, she said, "Oh. Wait a minute."

She was gone for a moment, then back on the phone:

"He just walked in."

She told me that Linda, the activities director, grabbed Mike as he walked in and sat him down at the piano. She would keep him playing until I get back.

When I walked into the big lobby, there was Mike pounding out "The Yellow Rose of Texas," Linda standing behind him with her hands firmly planted on his shoulders. Another resident was leaning against her walker, listening. When he finished the song, I told him I'd been looking for him. He folded his music book and followed me down the hall to the elevator. Even though it was cool outside, his shirt was drenched in sweat.

"Where've you been?"

"Well, I was at Pasquale's, but Jeannie and Bill never showed up!" he said, his voice too loud for the enclosed elevator.

"We're not meeting them until 6," I said.

"Well, I waited, but they never showed up. It was bizarre!"

"Did you go inside?"

"I had a cheese calzone and a glass of red wine."

"Really? How was it?"

"I don't know. They were closed."

"It was early," I told him.

"I went back and they were still closed!"

Had he walked to and from the restaurant twice, along busy Fair Oaks, part of the time in the dark? About half the time what Mike said was grossly inaccurate, and about half the time it was true, so there was no way of knowing what his past two and a half hours had been like. What I did know was that he absolutely should never be left alone again.

I felt as if I, too, was fast approaching a life behind locked walls and gates.

DAY CARE OR . . . ?

November 2010

U nder the guise that they needed a piano player and other help with their coming Christmas program, I got Mike set up on a twice a week day care program at Citrus Heights Bridges. Both Carol Kinsel of Senior Care Solutions and a woman in the dementia support group I sometimes attended said good things about this facility. That would provide two days a week of safety and activity for Mike, and two days a week for me to focus on other aspects of our lives that needed attention, and maybe even eke out a little reading time.

Citrus Heights Bridges was by far the most inviting of all the memory care facilities I'd recently visited. Even so, "most inviting" still didn't look all that good. I managed to keep Mike going there for nearly three weeks, but with each visit it became increasingly more difficult to get him out of our apartment and into the car as he kept insisting that he wasn't going to "that other convalescent home" ever again.

Each time I repeated what had now become a script: I can't absolutely, always, be with you. It's no longer safe for you to be left on your own. If you forget where I am, you might take off on foot, on a busy street, in search of me. That would be dangerous. Mike didn't contradict any of that. He simply kept repeating that he was not going to that awful place, and that the people there were uninteresting.

On Mike's sixth scheduled day at Citrus Heights Bridges, our 20-minute trip up there was miserable. He at first was asking that I let him out so he could walk home, then, with his hand on the door handle, telling me, "I'm getting out here." This at 60 miles an hour on I-80. I had the child lock on, but it still felt like risky business.

The director greeted Mike warmly when I walked him through the front door. "I'm so glad you're here," she said.

Mike's public persona kicked in.

"I'm happy to be here!"

When I picked him up at 2 in the afternoon, both the director and activities coordinator said how helpful he'd been in rehearsals for their upcoming Christmas program. They hoped Mike could help them out again, day after tomorrow.

"I'll be here!" he said, all smiles.

When we got in the car to go back to Carmichael Oaks Mike told me he hated Citrus Heights Bridges, he was never going back again, I couldn't make him go back again, and on and on. On the day of the next scheduled visit he was adamant about not going and refused to get dressed.

Shortly after I gave up on Citrus Heights Bridges, I heard that Rachel (mine for life) was now the director of The Guiding Star memory care facility, which was part of Porto Sicuro, a larger compound in Cameron Park that included luxurious condominiums for both independent and assisted living residents. I was surprised to learn that she'd left Riverside, but glad to know where she was currently working.

The leader of the dementia support group, as well as Carmichael Oaks staff and others who saw Mike often, all either directly or subtly, raised the issue of Mike's increasing difficulty. Some urged me to get prepared for the next step.

I'd been visiting local memory care facilities, knowing that the day would come when I would have to move Mike to such a place. Because Cameron Park was 30 miles from my home base, and because it looked quite luxurious, I'd not even considered a visit to that facility. But, remembering how effective Rachel had been with Mike, I decided to take a look.

I was again impressed with Rachel's empathy and understanding of dementia sufferers. The Guiding Star was in transition from one owner to the next and had many vacancies. As a result, it was less expensive than most other places I'd visited—a mere $2,800 monthly base fee, as compared to a minimum of $4,000 elsewhere. The Guiding Star at Porto Sicuro was also arranged in a way that felt less closed in than most other places. After a tour and a long conversation with Rachel, I decided to try Mike in The Guiding Star day program, once past the holidays. I completed the necessary paperwork that qualified Mike as either a part-time or a full-time resident. He could come for just a day, or two, or he could come to stay.

A few weeks after I'd completed the paperwork for Mike's entry to Porto Sicuro's Guiding Star unit, I drove back out to Cameron Park for one of Rachel's weekly dementia support group meetings. Since I was the only one who'd shown up for the "group" that day, I had a chance to talk more with Rachel about Mike. She was very certain of her methods and spoke of them with an almost missionary zeal. But her approach sounded more enlightened and humane than the ways in which I'd seen other caregivers deal with dementia charges. Not that I'd witnessed any brutality or unkindness, or neglect. My sense was that everyone was doing the best they could. But others seemed to lack the insight and intuition that Rachel exhibited. I was, though, concerned about what I had learned after her departure from Riverside, that Rachel moved around a lot.

"How long do you expect to be here at The Guiding Star?" I asked.

Rachel paused thoughtfully before answering. "Well, I'm a rolling stone," she said.

"Are you ready to roll?"

She laughed. "No. You don't need to worry about that. I got rid of everyone in this place when I took over here. I've hired only inexperienced caregivers, and I'm personally training each one. By the time I leave this place, it will be humming along like a well-tuned machine."

I left thinking that when the time came, this would be the place for Mike. I didn't know when that time would be.

In the meantime, I occasionally hired caregivers when things came up that I needed to attend to without Mike. Sometimes hired caregivers worked well, sometimes not. Friends and family continued to give me a break by taking Mike out for lunch, or to a movie, but his growing tendency to suddenly vanish from sight meant that an outing that was once manageable for one person now took two—one to buy the movie ticket or pay the restaurant bill, and another to race after Mike while the first person waited for change. Or one to wait at the table for the check while the other stood outside the restroom door, ready to guide Mike away from the exit and back to the table.

Our family Thanksgivings had, for decades, been celebrated with the Reynolds-Kyle family in their Woodacre home. It was an event we had both long enjoyed, and Mike was eager to get there. For several days before we were to leave he had been up before 6 asking, "Shall we go now?"

"Not today," I would tell him, and then tell him again, and again, and again. And I would tell myself, "It's not his fault. It's not his fault," again and again and again. That mantra, the serenity prayer, compartmentalizing worry, reading, help from friends and family, all helped me hang onto my goodwill and sanity. But the goodwill/sanity rope was fraying.

Finally, Tuesday morning around 10, worn down with trying to keep Mike focused on something besides leaving, we left for Woodacre. We'd just gotten on the freeway when Mike said we had to stop. He had to go to the bathroom.

"You just went before we left home," I reminded him.

"I have to go to the bathroom!" he said, reaching for the child-locked handle on the passenger side of the car.

"Okay. Let's find a gas station." I moved into the right lane for the next exit, running through my mind gas stations I knew to be close by.

Within minutes I pulled into the parking area of a Chevron station. I released the child lock, and Mike bolted out the door.

Once on our way again, Mike reclined his seat back as far as it would go and went to sleep.

The plan had been for us to get to Sharon and Doug's around 5 in the evening, in time for a light dinner. It generally took us two hours or less to make the 100-mile drive to their home in the woods above San Rafael. If I were lucky, we might hit a little traffic, extend the drive for an hour. Maybe I'd purposely take a wrong turn when I got to the fork that led one way toward San Rafael, the other toward Sonoma. Maybe we'd have lunch at that little Portuguese restaurant that we loved. I remembered that it was right there on the Plaza, easy to find. I remembered the potato soup that was more than potato soup, a Portuguese specialty.

I glanced over at the sleeping man who still looked a lot like Mike but wasn't. What was I thinking? When the opportunity to take the Sonoma turnoff appeared, I drove on by. I did take a Novato turn-off and drove aimlessly around for 30 or 40 minutes, then got back on the freeway headed toward Sharon and Doug's. I stopped for lunch at a familiar diner in San Anselmo, only 20 minutes or so from Woodacre. Mike ate quickly. "Let's go," he said.

I led him into a nearby specialty shop, with dinnerware and vases, handmade pottery and wall hangings. The man who'd loved to browse such places, loved to shop, stood in the doorway, scanned the room, and made a beeline back to the car. 1:45.

Before I pulled out from our parking space, I called Sharon.

"We're way early," I said. "I'm sorry."

"That's fine. The house is unlocked. I'll be home around 4, also."

"Okay."

"The downstairs is cleaned up and ready for you."

"Thanks."

"Hard morning?" she asked.

"Not really. Dad was in a huge hurry to leave home, though."

"Make yourselves at home. I'll see you a little later. The girls will probably be home around 4, also."

A few miles out of San Anselmo, on Sir Frances Drake Boulevard, the road became gently curvy, with a slight but steady incline and rolling hills on either side. At the turnoff to Woodacre, we entered a densely forested area with signs to watch for deer. We turned off the highway at the little Woodacre Market, a store that catered to the organic, gluten-free, raw foods, sometimes Paleo residents, and also to hikers and campers on their way to Samuel P. Taylor park and other, more distant campsites.

Just a few more blocks, then a steep and less-than-gentle curvy drive past Spirit Rock, then a sharp turn onto an even steeper driveway leading to Sharon and Doug's place. Another 60 feet or so and a sharp right, another steep incline, though for only about 20 feet, to a wide, level parking space, probably big enough for 10 or so cars if no one cared about being blocked in.

Their place was split level with a downstairs apartment where we often stayed when we visited. We carried our things down the driveway, then down the steps that led to the apartment. Once we unloaded, I led Mike upstairs to the living room where there was a TV. I found an old movie for him and went back downstairs hoping for a short nap. That worked for a little while.

For the past three years, our custom had been to spend the Tuesday night before Thanksgiving in Woodacre, so we could show up to Subei's Grandparents' Day at Marin Academy on Wednesday morning. Wednesday evening we'd have a simple dinner with just the 6 of us. Thanksgiving Day, Dale, Marg, and Corry would join us for the feast. Friday would be a movie day, then home on Friday evening.

This year, on Tuesday, just shortly after dinner with Sharon and Doug, Subei and Lena, Mike pushed away from the table, stood, and said, "Let's go home."

I reminded him of Grandparents' Day, and then Thanksgiving.

"Okay," he said. "I'll just go to bed," which he did.

The next morning, Wednesday, before 6, Mike was up. He had his jacket on over his pajamas. "Let's go home," he said.

"Not yet."

"I'll just wait for you in the car," he said, walking toward the door.

"No. Let's get dressed and we'll see if there's coffee upstairs."

"Okay," he said, putting on his shoes and walking up the driveway. "I'll wait for you in the car."

I followed behind, calling him back. With as much enthusiasm as I could muster, I suggested, "Let's have a cup of coffee before we leave."

Over the course of the next hour, I led him back from the driveway to exchange his pajama tops for a shirt, led back to exchange his pajama bottoms for pants, to shave, to brush his teeth and, finally, back up the driveway to the car.

At Marin Academy, a private high school with an enrollment of 400, 100 per class, there was a mix and mingle time in the lobby of the small but state-of-the-art theatre, with a nice spread of baked goods, and coffee or tea. Then we gathered on a beautiful patio where on one side there was a corner set up for students and their grandparents to have their pictures taken together, and on the other side tables where grandparents were given programs and a schedule of the classes we were to attend with our grandkids.

Mike spotted our 15-year-old-granddaughter, Subei. He greeted her with a big hug, and told her how happy he was to be there. We had our pictures taken, then went to our first classroom "assignment."

At Marin Academy, in a free and open setting, with just the right balance of guidance, Subei's creativity has blossomed. She's literally found her voice as a singer and enjoyed a freer approach to music than she previously experienced with formal piano and cello lessons. She's in an intellectually stimulating, and challenging, environment. It was delightful to meet her teachers and friends—a close-knit group of bright, funny, creative, caring teens.

Having taught for decades at a public alternative high school, though, I'm aware of the vast differences in educational opportunities for kids from affluent families and those from families living in, or near, the poverty level. I want Marin Academy quality of education for every kid, not just for my grandkids and their peers.

I stewed about the gross inequalities in our nation for a few moments, then led Mike to Room 207, where we would be exposed to Astrophysics with Subei in her second period class.

From the classroom presentations to music/dance performances in the theater, Mike followed my lead without complaint. The final event of the day took place in the gymnasium, with grandparents, friends and staff crowded onto the bleachers.

From my place in the bleachers, about 10 rows up, I noticed a strikingly attractive woman walking toward our section. She was wearing a brightly colored, free flowing garment, augmented with silky scarves of harmonizing colors. Her hair was thick and full and fell in long dreadlocks way past her shoulders. What a presence. Unlike me, who, in order to maintain my balance, practically had to crawl on hands and knees up to a vacant space in the bleachers, she stood straight and tall, taking her place just in front of us in two long strides.

Students, essentially the whole school, were crowded onto the court, participating in choral and dance presentations, performing both instrumental and vocal solo performances, and offering a few "spoken word" interpretations of their own, or someone else's, poetry. Between performances were group presentations of appreciation to staff and to fellow students. It was all very touching and captured my full attention.

Something, some slight stirring perhaps, shifted my attention to Mike. There he sat, holding one of the woman's long, tightly twisted dreadlocks between his thumb and index finger, rolling it back and forth.

"No, Mike!" I whispered, gently releasing the dreadlock to fall back into its rightful place. The woman didn't stir, but it was just one more sign that the part of Mike's brain that inhibits inappropriate behavior was losing ground.

The rest of our visit was, "Let's go. Let's go. Let's go."

A few days after our return from Woodacre, back at Carmichael Oaks, we were in the elevator on our way to dinner. It stopped, for no apparent reason, on the second floor. The doors opened and Mike stepped forward. I touched his arm. "Not yet," I told him. "We want the first floor."

He turned toward me, then stomped to the back of the elevator—the Carmichael Oaks elevators are big enough to accommodate wheelchairs. Big enough to stomp in.

Mike stood straight and stiff at the back, scowling.

"You seem so angry," I said.

This was simply an observation, stated calmly.

Head thrust forward, fists clenched, Mike shouted, "I AM ANGRY! I FEEL LIKE SMACKING YOU!!"

In the blink of an eye a whole array of possibilities appeared before me. I saw myself standing close to him, challenging him. "YOU WOULDN'T DARE SMACK ME!" I might say, taking the hit. That would start the ball rolling. A call to the police. A 72-hour observation period. A placement decision. How easy that could be?

Instead I said, calmly, "Smacking me wouldn't be a good idea."

"Why? What would happen?" he said.

"I would be out of here so fast it would make your head spin. I don't know who would take care of you then, but it wouldn't be me."

Whether or not Mike got what I said is uncertain, but he was unusually subdued for the rest of the evening.

Not long after that incident I took Mike with me to the Folsom Toyota dealer to get our car serviced. He sat with me in the office while the service manager wrote the repair order, then went with me into the lobby area where we were to wait for the shuttle to take us back home. No sooner had we sat down than Mike stood up again.

"Let's go!"

"We're waiting for the shuttle," I said. "Let's get some coffee from the machine."

That took about three minutes.

"Let's go get the car," Mike said.

"It won't be ready until this afternoon."

"I'll just walk home," he said.

"Mike. You can't walk home. It's pouring down rain, and we're 10 miles away from home."

"I'll just walk."

"No. Look at those stuffed animals over there. Do you think Mika would like one?"

"Let's rent a car."

"The shuttle will be here soon."

"We should just go buy a car."

"Our car will be fine as soon as it's serviced."

"Okay. I'm walking!"

He rushed toward the door, then, miracle of miracles, a longtime friend came walking through the door Mike was about to leave by.

"Dave Dawson!" Mike said, his old social self emerging.

"Well, if it isn't the Reynoldses," Dave said. "I suppose you're out on this stormy morning for the same reason I am."

"Mike was just threatening to walk home," I said, careful to keep my tone light.

Dave, who knew of Mike's situation, said, "Oh, you don't want to do that. Let's get some of that free coffee over there."

"Sure," Mike said, following Dave to the coffee cart.

A few minutes later we were called for the shuttle.

Once back in the apartment, I turned on the TV and found an old movie for Mike to watch. That held his attention for about 10 minutes, after which he turned off the TV.

"Let's go get the car," he said.

"It's not time yet. They'll call us."

That was the theme for the next four hours. Mike's agitation increased. His attention span decreased. And this day was undoubtedly better than the next would be.

March 2015

Dear Mike,

Flipping through one of the journals you left behind, journals that had been boxed up since we left Gold River, I read, "I've made a terrible mistake. I hope Marilyn never, ever learns of this."

You wrote this when you were on a music fellowship in Vienna, in the fall of 1985. You would have been 45.

I think back to that time, wondering what your terrible mistake might have been. Would this have been one of those secrets that one sometimes hears about, of a widowed/ widowered (?) spouse's discovery that somehow shatters the very foundations of the marriage they thought they'd had, that destroys so much of their understanding of who they had been in the world, with their partner, that now every single thing about their life is called into question? Would this have been one of those revelations that destroys one's very sense of identity, sweeps it all away, like some fragile leaf tumbled and torn apart in a storm? I can't imagine what that would be. Whatever it was, you must have thought of it as a betrayal. Was it an affair with some woman? A man? I felt certain whatever it was didn't involve theft, or murder, or a hit and run in a rented car.

In my memory, those years of the '80s were good years for us. In 1985, Matt was 16, playing club soccer, doing well-enough in high school. Sharon and Cindi were in their 20s, Sharon in Northern California, studying to become a chiropractor, Cindi newly married and living in Massachusetts where her then-husband was stationed. With just the three of us at home, our lives were less complicated and demanding than when all five us lived under the same roof.

You'd been nominated for LA County Music Teacher of the Year. As tenor soloist at All Saints you were musically and spiritually both challenged and, mostly, fulfilled. My first published essay appeared in the Los Angeles Times in the early '80s. Together we'd completed a three-month course at the Pritikin Center in Santa Monica that led us to a much more healthy lifestyle than we'd developed, or fallen into, in our years together. For the first time ever, your cholesterol was in a normal range. Money was not nearly as tight as it once had been. We enjoyed weekend getaways together, mini-honeymoons of sorts. During that time we probably argued over choices of paint color, or wallpaper, or how to handle Matt's consistent refusal to honor our curfew expectations. We could always fall back on money if we were looking for an argument. You wanting to charge a new item of furniture, or a suit, or a trip, me wanting to hold off until we could pay cash. Truly, though, because we kept most of our money separate, these arguments were not rancorous. There was no rancor between us.

So, 1985. I was tempted to start at the beginning of that Vienna journal, read it all the way through, try to ferret out the source of your shame. But why? You hadn't wanted me to know. Did I need to know?

My best guess is that you and our opera singer friend, Rosalie, "slept" together one or more times during your stay in Vienna. You loved each other in the way that close friends can, sharing thoughts about books, and music, and the wealth of joys and fears inherent to performing singers. Vowel placement, breath control, care of the cherished throat and vocal chords—such conversations were fascinating and precious to you and Rosalie. Just as you were not either capable or willing to talk at length about the advantages of first person vs. third person point of view in a piece of fiction, I was not up for lengthy discussions of tongue placement in maintaining open vowels. There is a particular intimacy in one's sharing talk about something dear to them, but not so dear to most others. Maybe your platonic intimacy crossed a line?

Enough conjecture. Your letters home during that time expressed your delight at being in Vienna, steeped in music, enjoying new musician friends. You also wrote of your extreme longing and loneliness for me. On your return from Vienna, if I'd learned what you didn't want me to know, we might have needed a few sessions with a marriage counselor. We would not have needed a divorce lawyer.

I was more puzzled by your need to keep a secret than by the secret itself. Was it shame? Did you not trust me?

At one point, just before your FTD diagnosis but long after symptoms had arisen, you told me you didn't feel safe with me. I remember we were sitting at the breakfast bar in the Promontory Point kitchen. We were each on our second cup of coffee, the newspaper spread out before us. I don't remember any of the conversation leading up to this, but I remember very distinctly the tightness of your face and voice as you announced, "I don't feel safe with you."

I was stunned! How could that be? Since the very beginning I'd loved you, unwaveringly, with all my heart. I'd loved you for who you were, considered you, us, in everything I did. How could you not feel safe with me? When I asked that question, you simply answered, "I just don't."

I know now, at least I think I know now, that frontotemporal dementia had already begun messing with your emotions, your stability, your capacity for reasoning. But if it was FTD then, what was it in 1985 that caused you to feel a need to build a wall around your secret? Were there other walls?

I picked up another journal, this one from the later '80s. You'd written of how much you loved me, how you loved seeing me grow as a writer. How you wanted to be as supportive of my writing as I had always been of your singing.

You'd written of everyday things, taking Matt to soccer practice at the Rose Bowl. You remembered that, on one of your father's December visits from Florida, you'd taken him to that area around the Rose Bowl where the two of you watched all manner of people readying floats for the big day. You sometimes still missed your father. We'd been to Nancy Obrien's for dinner and laughed ourselves silly over the stories D.D. told about tuning Frank Sinatra's rat turd-infused Steinway.

Reading your entry, I was so lonesome for you, for your voice, your phrases, your distinct take on things, that I wanted to devour every word you'd written in every journal you'd ever kept. But what if there were more secrets? And what if other people came across them after my death? In spite of a hunger for your words, a hunger that bordered on pain, I could not disrespect your written secrets. I could not disrespect the secrets that might fall into other hands after my death. I did what I knew you would want me to do. I destroyed your journals.

Into a heavy-duty trash bag, I first poured a few cups of water, then dropped your journal with the recently revealed secret into the bag. All of the journals were good quality, with heavy covers, quality paper, and tightly bound pages. (You always appreciated quality.) To pull each journal apart and shred the pages was more of a task than I cared to undertake. So enough water to be absorbed by journal pages, and on top of that sour milk that had been sitting in the refrigerator since Matt and Mika returned home from last month's visit. Then a little more water, another journal, something else rotten from the refrigerator. Obviously, I'd been needing to clean out the refrigerator for quite some time. I established a rhythm—a little more water, a journal, something rotten from the refrigerator. A little more water, a journal, something rotten from the refrigerator, etc., etc., etc. With the last journal resting underneath a sea of slimy lettuce, I half-carried, half-dragged the trash bag to the backyard. For good measure, I heaved two shovels full of dirt into the bag before pulling the ties into a tight knot. Careful to lift with my legs, I hoisted the whole mess into the city's big, grey, plastic container and secured the lid.

I stood staring at the receptacle of your words, feeling that now familiar sense of emptiness that comes with the everyday reminders of losses, both big and little, of your absence from the world and from me. I did what I sometimes do now, during an afternoon of sadness. I stretched out on the bed with my iPad and took up where I'd left off reading my current book, The Little Red Chairs *by Edna O'Brien. But as compelling as that story was, my mind kept going back to secrets.*

I'd been so puzzled by your need to keep a secret from me, that I'd nearly forgotten secrets I'd kept from you. For what? For your own protection? To spare myself embarrassment? Many years ago, there was the nearly innocent, more than friends, relationship with a teaching colleague of mine. There'd been details from the lives of our kids that I knew about but didn't pass on to you. I'd never lied about any of this, but I'd chosen to keep certain things to myself. Things that I knew would anger you I kept to myself. Things that I knew would hurt you I kept to myself. My guess is that the same was true for you. For most of our married life, the secrets I kept from you were few and far apart. Again, my guess is that the same was true for you.

With the onslaught of FTD, my keeping secrets, my outright lies to you, became so prevalent that I feared the time would come when I wouldn't know truth from fiction. There were the lies about damage to our house that forced us to live in Carmichael Oaks, the lies that that move was only temporary, the lies that I was going to meet a teacher friend to work on a project when really, I was sneaking over to our old house to continue the emptying it of the contents leftover from the basics I'd had moved to Carmichael Oaks. Thousands of everyday lies until the final, that worst lie of all. Assuring you that I'd be back to pick you up after lunch, after leaving you at the securely locked memory care facility in Cameron Park. My heart aches even now, five years later, to remember that day. To remember that lie.

But we'd started with secrets, hadn't we? That you'd felt it necessary to keep a secret from me was a slight surprise. Nothing more. It did not shake my understanding of who we had been in the world, or cause me to call our whole marriage into question, or destroy my sense of identity. Had you been the one left on earth after I was ashes in the ocean, I suspect that the same would have been true for you, had you discovered a secret in one of my journals. I suspect that you would have wanted to read whatever journal you could find, longing for my words, my voice. Would you have ended up depositing my journals into a trash bag, mixing them with water and rotten food, and dumping them?

It's strange—these letters. These speculations. I'm having "conversations" with you that I need to have, ones I can't have with anyone else in the world. As I write to the missing you, it's as if you are there, somewhere, listening—a consoling illusion.

Missing you still,
Marilyn

WHAT WE ALL KNEW

December 2010

Christmas was a repeat of Thanksgiving, only more so. Mike wanted to leave for Sharon and Doug's days ahead of time, then about 15 minutes into the drive, Christmas Eve day, asked, "When are we coming back home?"

After the opening of gifts that evening, probably around 8, Mike announced he was going to bed. I followed him out to the outside "shack" that had been converted into a guest room. I wanted to be sure he could find his pajamas. He took his shoes off and crawled into bed. I got his pajamas from the suitcase and suggested he put them on.

"I want to go home," he said.

"No. We're staying through Christmas. We'll go home the day after Christmas, like we always do…. Here, you'll be more comfortable in these," I said, placing his pajamas at the foot of the bed.

He put them on, crawled back in bed, asked to go home.

I again told him we were staying through Christmas.

"I'll just walk home then," he said, getting out of bed and reaching for the door.

I moved in front of the door.

"No, Mike. We're spending the night."

"I'll just stay in bed then!" he said, throwing back the covers. "I know how to do that!"

He got back into bed, yanked the covers over him, and turned his back to me.

I went back to join the rest of the family. Within minutes Mike was back in the house asking to go home. This routine continued throughout our stay, becoming even more incessant than it had at Thanksgiving. He was miserable. I was miserable. And although everyone carried on with the festivities, the contrast between Mike's present constant state of anxiety and his joyous holiday personality of Christmases past was terrible to witness.

When it was finally time to say our goodbyes and drive away, we all knew without a doubt that Mike had spent his last Christmas with us. The husband who had, with such energy and enthusiasm, decorated the house to the hilt and lit up the whole outside, the grampa who had carefully wrapped gifts and signed tags from Mr. Claus, or the Christmas Fairy, or Rudolph, who had bought extravagant Christmas outfits for each of the grandkids for as long as they would go along with it, the dad who chose gifts with care and collaborated with grown-up cooks on food and drinks, the brother-in-law who every Christmas made an over-the-top extravagantly fancy birthday dessert, the singer whose holiday season was frantically busy with church programs and caroling gigs—that man was gone. He was gone. He wasn't coming back. Whether we said it or not, we all knew.

The day after we returned from Woodacre, I called Porto Sicuro and arranged with Rachel to move Mike into their Guiding Star memory care section. While the activities director kept Mike occupied with the weekly sing-along, I rushed out to Best Buy and bought a basic TV for the private room, sheets for the extra long single bed, and a comforter. On December 29, 2011, I drove Mike the 20 miles to Cameron Park.

It was time. It was past time.

THIS IS MY FATHER'S WORLD

December 29, 2010

After my call to The Guiding Star, I contacted the senior relocation service that had helped with our move to the Carmichael Oaks apartment. I arranged to have Mike's room set up, ready and waiting with familiar pictures and furnishings. Two days later, mid-morning, I told Mike I was taking him to a new place where he could play the piano and entertain the residents.

"I'm not going back to that place," he said, referring to the Citrus Heights Bridges memory care program where I'd tried to get him set up on a Tuesday/Thursday schedule.

"This is a different place. Rachel's there. Remember Rachel?"

"Yes. I'm not going."

But he did go. He followed me to the car and got in. On the freeway he asked numerous times to be let out so he could walk home.

Dale had earlier burned a CD for me of instrumental arrangements of hymns. We both loved the old Baptist hymns we'd grown up with, though we'd long ago rejected the accompanying theology. The wordless instrumentals were perfect, though in reality the music wasn't wordless. The words were all lying dormant in my mind, brought to the surface by the old, familiar tunes.

I started the CD, hoping it might have a calming effect on Mike.

"Do you like the music?" I asked.

"Yes," he said. He sat quietly, seeming to listen, then breaking the spell to ask, "You're not going to leave me there, are you?"

He asked that many times, and many times I answered with a lie. "I'll pick you up this afternoon," I always said.

I followed the experts' advice for dealing with dementia sufferers: Keep it simple. Be reassuring. Don't try to explain because they can't understand. Explanations will only further confuse them. Tell the kindest story. Lies, lies, desperate lies.

Rachel met us at the front door, quickly managing to charm Mike as she'd done at their first meeting. She spoke simply and gently, saying she could use his help. Could he help her a little? Maybe play the piano for a while and talk with residents?

"Sure!" Mike said, answering with his old enthusiasm.

I kissed him goodbye, told him I'd see him soon, and walked to the door. He followed along, but Rachel easily led him back toward her office.

By the time I made it to the circular driveway that led past The Guiding Star entrance, Mike was standing close against the glass entrance doors. He watched, forlorn, as I drove away. The CD automatically started again. Of all hymns to land on it was "This is My Father's world…" and to my listening ears/ all nature sings/and round me rings the music of the spheres….

And there he was, suddenly before me, the young Mike, in his blue choir robe, gracefully, magically, drawing music from a disparate group of children, my own among them—Sharon, 8, Cindi, 7, eyes glued to the man who was, unbeknownst to any of us, soon to become their father. The song continues, "I rest me in the thought of rocks and trees, of skies and seas/His hand the wonders wrought…."

The nearly 40 good years with Mike overcame the past few bad years, and a torrential flood of long blocked sobs burst through. I pulled to the side of the road, weeping for all that was lost to me, and even more for all that was lost to Mike, and for those two now-grown little girls, and for the son who came later, and for the dog, and the lost house, and for wars and famines and every other damned sorrow in the world, and then back to Mike, back to those scenes of who he had been and of who he had become.

Who knows how long I sat there? Finally the wrenching sobs subsided, and my focus shifted to the present. To tasks at hand, to what was next. I found a crumpled Starbucks napkin in the glove compartment, wiped my face and blew my nose, took five deep yoga breaths and deemed myself fit to drive.

As I turned onto the freeway, heading back to Sacramento, dark clouds parted to reveal a growing patch of sunny blue sky. If this were a movie, or a novel, such a scene would be trite and contrived. But it was neither of those. It was my life. And, knowing there would be more darkness to come, I treasured the fleeting gift of light.

GRIEF STOPS BY

Me: What? Yeah, you can visit for a while. But I can't see you very well. Come in out of the shadows … Wait. Who else is with you?

Grief: My family. My father Death; Mother Loss; Sister Disease; Brother Injustice; Cousins Anger, Disappointment, Regret, Resentment …

I only invited you.

We stick together—me and my family.

Well … come on in. You can come through the living room, but if this is an overnight, you'll have to stay in the back room.

The back room? I deserve a better place than your dusty old back room. Why can't I stay in your living room?

I prefer other company.

You can't pretend I don't exist. You can't ignore me. If you ignore me, there will be repercussions with the Cousins, maybe even with Sister.

Don't threaten me. I'm not ignoring you. I'm simply keeping you where you belong. You don't get to be free range in my domicile. You're only in the living room for a short conversation, because I invited you.

What about your precious Joy? She gets to come and go as she pleases.

I like her better. I prefer Joy to Grief.

You can't truly know Joy without knowing Grief.

Maybe, but since I know both, I prefer Joy.

I always get a bum rap.

Not really. Plenty of people prefer you to Joy. You make them feel important. They let you be queen of their domicile. I'm not one of them.

You have to admit that I have influence, though. Like the other evening at Kathy's party, or when you wake up in the middle of the night and find me in bed with you.…

Yes, there are times when you loom large. Kathy's party, celebrating her 70 years of life, telling stories of our decades of friendship and shared work. Suddenly you shoved your way in, forcing me to feel the emptiness that is Mike's absence. The pure tenor voice, absent from the "Happy Birthday," song. The silly, animated version of Mike's famous party hokey-pokey, absent. In the midst of warmth and laughter, you and emptiness were, momentarily, my only reality.

It's taken a long time for you to recognize me. When your father died, I couldn't even get through the door, much less find a place in your living room.

I was busy with the cousins—Anger, Disappointment, Abandonment....

You had all those armed guards around your place—special instructions to keep me out.

Yes. Well, it turned out I had to banish the guards. They were arming for a hostile takeover and … Hey! Hey! What are you doing?

Unpacking. The guards are gone.

No, you don't! Out of the living room. You've been here long enough for one day. And take your family with you! You've got way bigger jobs to do. Make your way to the people who are sick and hungry, to the ones fighting wars, the ones being tortured and abused. My grief is petty in comparison. Out!

Have it your way. But I'll be back. You can count on that!

I know. You are always hovering, waiting for that moment when the door opens and you can rush in.

Yep. And don't sell me short. I have many keys to that door—the smell of morning coffee, the red wool jacket still hanging in the closet, the morning surprise that the warm body you wake to is only a dog. So many keys to the door.

Yes, but you'll have to keep the visits short.

MY LIFE
AS A NOMAD
January through July 2011

Without Mike, I have no need or desire to live in a three-tiered retirement community. As much as I appreciated Carmichael Oaks as a port in the storm, I'm eager to move on. Also, because of the $3,000-plus rent, I need to get out of here as soon as possible.

As I busy myself with packing, separating the necessities to keep with me from things to be stored, wherever, until I decide where I'll be for the longer term, as I wait in the checkout line at Raley's, as I drift off to sleep at night and waken to reality in the morning, there's the overpowering image of Mike pacing round and round, behind locked doors, a caged tiger, poised to bolt, an image more real than the groceries in the basket, the cheerful cashier asking about my day, the debit card I'm pulling from my purse.

First thing in the morning, last thing at night, pre-dawn times of wakefulness, all day, every day, Mike caged. Mike rushing the door. Mike peering out, watching for the Prius, for me, to pull up to the curb and come to him. I am haunted. Tortured. How could I do that to him, essentially put him in prison? How could I not? What else might I have done? Over and over the images, the questions, the indescribable ache of emptiness in the center of my being. All day. All night. Every day. Every night. Us separated. Mike caged.

It seemed necessary to have my phone on and within reach at all times, in case of an emergency call, but after the first week or so I stopped answering Mike's nighttime calls. During the day I took to answering only one out of every two or three calls from Mike. That still left me hearing his come-get-me-fuck-you mantra 10 to 15 times a day.

Rachel advised that, since I was a "trigger," I not visit Mike until he'd become better adjusted to life at The Guiding Star. Other friends and family visited. Mike was happy to see them. Joe and Kathy lived just a few miles from The

Guiding Star and often dropped by for a quick visit when they were on their way to the market, or Home Depot, or any number of places that took them right past Porto Sicuro. If the weather was nice when they visited, they'd take Mike for a walk around the grounds. When it was time for them to leave, he willingly returned to The Guiding Star with them. Once inside, one of the caregivers would distract him while they were "buzzed out." Marg, Dale, Judy, Jo, others of the 100 Hours Club all visited Mike before I did.

Friends and family called Mike on his cell. He greeted them happily, responded to questions. How was he? Fine. Was he playing the piano? Yes. How was the food? Good. He didn't initiate conversation, but he maintained his old cheerful phone persona. As far as I know, the only original remark he made in any phone call was when, after two weeks at The Guiding Star, he told Matt quite matter of factly, "Your mother divorced me."

Though his brain had lost all capacity for logic and reasoning, his intuition was still at work. I had not, in fact, divorced him, but neither had I been his wife for some time. My recent roles with Mike had been closer to mother, financial conservator, caregiver and behavior monitor, none of which was conducive to a husband-wife relationship. It had probably been over a year since we'd gone through the motions of "making love," a euphemism for the kind of sex one may have with a partner who has lost the capacity to love. Who knows how long it had been since we'd actually made love? I hadn't been keeping track.

By the end of the first four weeks at The Guiding Star, Rachel felt that Mike was sufficiently adjusted to the move that I could visit. I took chocolate chip cookies from his favorite bakery, snapshots of the grandkids, a CD of Artur Rubenstein playing Chopin waltzes, and a few more clothes. I got there around 10 in the morning and found Mike sitting alone, expressionless, at a table in the dining room. He rose from his chair, smiling broadly, crossed the dining room and greeted me with a kiss.

"Let's go," he said.

"Can I see your room?"

He turned and walked quickly down the hall. I followed close behind. His room was neat, with the familiar pictures on the wall. A favorite lamp that had belonged to his great aunt was on one of our bedside tables that now sat beside

Mike's extra long twin.

"Look," I said, holding up the CD. "Shall we listen to some of the waltzes?"

"Let's go!" he said, walking quickly out the door and down the hall. I caught up with him at the entryway. He was carrying a leather picture album, the size of a paperback book, that contained family pictures and some loose postcards.

"Let's go!" he said, pushing at the thick glass door.

"Look, I brought some cookies. Can we get some coffee?"

He followed me into the dining room. I got coffee from the ever-present giant coffeemaker and took the cups to the table where I'd first seen him.

"Come sit down for a minute."

He did. I gave him a cookie. He downed it in two big bites, took a swallow of coffee and stood.

"Let's go!"

Rachel, who had been watching from a distance, came over to Mike and took his arm. "Can you please help me with some music?" she said, leading him toward the lobby piano.

I went to the door where an aide was waiting to let me out.

In the Prius, my face covered with my hands, my head leaning against the steering wheel, I sobbed. Poor Mike. Poor me. Goddamnitall!

Rachel and I were keeping in close touch through email and the evening after that first visit she wrote:

After you left, Mike became extremely agitated, shouted, stormed the door several times. We just got him calmed down. He is back to the behaviors of before the medication change. We need to ride this out to see if he settles down before any more visits. I don't want to have his meds adjusted just because of visitations.... It will take more adjustment time for him to acclimate to the routine. One day at a time.

It was another four weeks before I visited again. In the meantime Mike lost his cell phone. He could still call me, and did, but because he now had to use the phone in Rachel's office, his calls were less frequent. On the rare days when he didn't call me, I called him. Matt and Sharon called often.

During this time of separation I sent cards to Mike, sometimes including a family snapshot of better times. I posted his mailing address on the blog in case others wanted to drop him a line. I looked at rentals.

Mike's care used all of his retirement income and half of mine. At the rate I was cashing in our lessened-in-value IRAs and mutual funds, I had another year, at the most two years, during which I could meet basic expenses. Over the past year, I'd watched what had once seemed more than adequate retirement savings hemorrhage away. With the house in foreclosure and many credit card balances long overdue, our once pristine credit rating was in the sewer. Landlords were not eager to rent to me. Decent places within my perceived price range were rare.

I toured Vintage Woods Senior Apartments, an "affordable living" complex somewhere about halfway between Sacramento and Cameron Park. It had two bedrooms, one of which would work nicely for an office. It was freshly painted and carpeted, and there was a well-maintained pool and clubhouse. They accepted pets of 20 pounds or less. Sunny hovered around 18. The rent was low enough that I could almost cover Mike's expenses and still make ends meet. Because I would be left with so little discretionary income after paying for Mike's placement in a memory care facility, the manager of the complex was certain I would qualify. Credit scores were not a consideration.

There was one available apartment, upstairs, overlooking the courtyard. The rooms were not spacious, but I knew it could easily work for my pared-down life. The design was such that even though the rooms were small, the apartment felt light and open.

I pictured myself living there. The complex backed up to a large park, a perfect place to walk Sunny. It was only a block to a Raley's market, my favorite Northern California chain. I pictured myself walking to and from the market, my portable rolling cart filled with the few weekly supplies necessary for my simplified life. I pictured myself reading by the pool. Playing Scrabble in the clubhouse. I pictured where the desk would go.

My application was turned down. I made an appointment with the manager's immediate supervisor but it was of no use. Our gross income was too much for me to qualify for a designated affordable senior apartment. The corporate contact person clarified that, yes, they did deduct valid medical expenses from gross income when evaluating whether or not a potential renter qualified as "low income." Unfortunately, costs related to memory care were not considered to be valid medical expenses.

Had Mike's disease been anything other than FTD—diabetes, or cancer, or heart disease or any of the other major killers of our time—his expenses would have been completely covered by our health insurance. If we'd had no health insurance coverage, the expenses related to such a disease would have been deducted from my gross income, thus meeting the low-income requirements of the affordable living complex. Not so with FTD.

There were other housing options. Matt and Leesa assured me that I would be more than welcome to stay with them in Walla Walla. We agreed it would be a good thing all around if I could be a regular part of Mika's life.

I couldn't picture myself living in Walla Walla, 900 miles from Mike in Cameron Park. As I weighed the possibility of such a move, I explored memory care facilities that might work for Mike. The two private facilities were dreary beyond description, but I was impressed with the Walla Walla Odd Fellows home. It offered independent living, assisted living, and nursing care. It was considerably less expensive than any places available in the Sacramento area. It was long established, with a friendly, caring staff and spacious, beautifully landscaped grounds. Just blocks from where Matt taught at Whitman College, and just a few more blocks from where they lived, Walla Walla had its appeal. The Odd Fellows didn't have a secure memory care facility. They had a buzzer system that alerted staff whenever anyone left the assisted living facility, but they were not set up to deal with residents with "exit-seeking behavior." If I chose to make a move, they were willing to give Mike a try in the hope that he would adapt within a month or so. But what were the chances that Mike would adapt? Slim to none was my guess. Then where would we be?

Another option was the downstairs apartment at Sharon and Doug's in Woodacre. One-bedroom with a nice-sized living room, a small but convenient kitchen, full bath, and large outdoor deck, it would easily accommodate my needs. Sharon and Doug assured me that I would be welcome there. As with the Walla Walla possibility, I would be happy to be a part of the grandkids' everyday lives. In both cases, Walla Walla or Woodacre, I could offer basic help to overburdened parents. Hanging out with Mika after school would be great fun. For Subei and Lena, hanging out with Gramma wasn't quite as exciting as it was to Mika, but they still liked me. I could still make them laugh. My greatest Woodacre asset would be providing taxi service, something I could happily do.

I needed to get out of Carmichael Oaks, but I didn't yet know where I would go.

I arranged for the moonlighting movers to move things from storage to Joe and Kathy's barn, then to move furniture from the apartment to storage. It seemed certain that I'd never again have a bedroom large enough for our Stickley furniture, so I had the bed delivered to a local furniture consignment store. One of the movers was happy to get the still relatively new king-sized mattress and box springs. The large chest and bedside tables were stored in the hope that they might someday fit into a new space.

In the Prius I kept Sunny's bed, food and dishes, a medium-sized suitcase packed with the essentials of a one-to two-week outing, including medications and cosmetics. My laptop was tucked out of sight under the passenger seat. There were two plastic hanging file containers, one with basic personal business necessities, bankruptcy papers, bills, tax information, insurance documents, Mike's medical records and the Porto Sicuro contract. The other file had basic book-business papers—an accepted proposal for an upcoming English teacher's conference, the Morning Glory Press contract for *Over 70 and I Don't Mean MPH,* and the nearly completed manuscript for that essay collection. A lightweight garment bag contained hanging clothes, mostly cottons.

I would be a nomad until I could settle on something more permanent.

August 2015

Dear Mike,

Sometimes I hear you calling my name—not frantically, but as if you want to draw attention to something. It's the way you called my name on thousands, tens of thousands, of occasions. Like that time way back in the '60s, when we were in Dr. Groat's office, getting blood tests for our marriage license. I'd already had my blood drawn and was walking down the hall to the exit when I heard, "Marilyn!"

It was almost a whisper, and I turned to see you sitting in an examination room, motioning to me. I expected you were going to point out something that was funny, maybe that standard picture of the uterus that so often adorns the walls of doctors' examining rooms. The one that includes ovaries, fallopian tubes, cervix and vagina. The one that looks like Bessie the Moo Cow. But instead of sharing something humorous, you said, "I think I'm going to faint." Your squeamishness at the sight of blood was another detail to add to my getting-to-know-you cup of characteristics.

You called my name when you woke me gently on mornings when you were already up and showered, ready for your zero period class. Or when, unlike in the doctor's office, you did draw my attention to something we could share a laugh over. Or when you caught my attention in a restaurant, or a party, or any number of places where, because of our unsynched schedules, we'd arrived separately.

At first, before I was used to you being gone, when I heard you call my name, I would turn instinctively, expecting to see you. That was years ago. Now, I just get quiet and listen, welcoming the memories that come with the unique tone and rhythm of your voice and my name.

This morning, at UUSS, we sang "Come, Thou Fount of Every Blessing." The singing of that familiar melody is just as rousing with the UUs as it was with the Baptists, but the words to the hymn have been adapted to UU sensibilities. Today's lyrics are much more in keeping with my own understanding and insights. Jesus and His blood are nowhere to be found in today's version. But at the beginning of the second verse, as the congregation sings, "Come, thou fount of every vision, lift our eyes to what may come ..." I shift back to the Christian hymnal version:

"Here I raise mine Ebenezer/Hither by Thy help I've come/And I hope, by Thy good pleasure/Safely to arrive at home...."

We were young. Well, at 28, you were young. At 33, I was young-ish. Dale and Marg at, what, 22? Maybe 23? They were definitely young. I don't remember when and where it was that the four of us got so silly over that song. What I do remember is that when we got to "Now I raise mine Ebenezer ..." you, with your comedic gestures and timing, glanced furtively down toward your "Ebenezer" and sang with gusto "... by Thy help I've come" and "... good pleasure ..." and "arrive at home," and forever after, that song transports me back to a time of shared laughter and silliness, and though some might interpret this as sacrilegious, to me it's a sacred joy. I doubt that whatever God there may be is offended.

I cherish memories of those times, Mike. I cherish hearing you call my name. I cherish memories of laughter. I cherish memories of your raised Ebenezer.

Marilyn

FEWER
OUTBURSTS
May 2011

Mike has had very few outbursts these past few weeks. That's a huge relief, even in the midst of my overwhelming sadness at Mike's present state of being. Are the lessened outbursts due to the tweaked and balanced drug regimen, or is he indeed adjusting to life at The Guiding Star? Who can say? Whatever the reason, I'm grateful.

During a three-week stay in the Reynolds-Kyle downstairs apartment, I managed to finish the semifinal draft of *Over 70 and I Don't Mean MPH*. Part of that time included keeping the Woodacre ship afloat while the others were on vacation. My duties were few—feed their elephant-sized dog and the bitchy cat, keep seed in the feeders for the hoard of ravenous birds that Sharon supports, and water a few plants. Easy-peasy.

The next stop in my nomadic route will be at the Dodsons', in time for their annual July Fourth KFC pig-out.

These days Mike is usually in bed when I visit. He doesn't want to associate with anyone at The Guiding Star, and so, other than meals, he takes to his bed. Now that he's less agitated, the caregivers take him out for a walk a few times a day, but that's about it.

A typical visit for me was on July 7. Mike was in bed when I got there. He was lying on his side, facing the door.

"Hi, Mike!" I said, smiling my most cheerful smile.

He brightened and said "hi." I did the usual, asking how he was. "Fine." What had he been doing? "Playing the piano." I gave him news of Sharon and her family, Matt and Mika, etc. He was blank, then turned with his back to me and faced the wall. I sat in the chair beside his bed and read the paper for a while. Mike appeared to be sleeping. I gave him a light kiss on the forehead and left. Thirty minutes out. Thirty minutes back. Twelve minutes there.

Dale and Marg visited a few days later. Mike was in the living room with the others, batting a big balloon-like ball around. They joined in, then the three of them went to "Mike's table" in the dining room where they each had a latte. In addition to being the hairstylist assistant, Marg generally brings lattes when she visits. Their report of this visit was that Mike was momentarily engaged when they talked of Marg's upcoming trip to Montana, then he was gone again.

Although Mike now usually gives one-word answers to questions and doesn't talk beyond that, he sometimes surprises me. On another July visit, Mike was in his room but got up when I suggested we go out to the patio. We sat for a short time while I tried to keep the chatter going.

"Shall we go inside?" Mike said.

I followed him into the dining room where we sat at his table. I had a bite of lunch with him, then left before he was finished. He stays fairly focused on food, so it was easy to leave without him trying to follow. But the question, "Shall we go inside?" was surprisingly clear and in context with the situation.

From what I can tell, Mike is more talkative with other visitors and staff than he is with me, though "talkative" is an exaggeration. With me he is mostly blank, though there are times when he sits watching me intently, waiting, I suspect, for me to take him "home."

On another July visit, Mike asked, "When do we go to the boat?"

I said I wasn't sure and asked what time he thought we should be there.

"Five o'clock," he said.

I told him that sounded about right, then took him out to the patio where I handed him the clippers and sat with him while he clipped his nails. It's quite a chore for him, though so far he gets the job done.

On the way home, processing the visit, I wondered about the boat remark. Earlier in the day I'd told Mike that his brother, Jerry, was coming to town soon. He gave no reaction to that news until I said, "It will be fun to see Jerry, won't it?"

"Yes," he'd said, but without affect.

But … some 30-plus years ago Mike, Matt and I joined Jerry, Jackie, and their son David for a Caribbean cruise. We flew into Miami and met Jerry and family at the ship. Did Mike jump from news of a visit from Jerry to that long ago cruise? To wondering when we needed to go to the boat? There's no making sense of any of it, but I can't help trying.

Besides Jerry, his three grown kids, Beth, Laura, and David, are also coming to see Mike. I'm eager to see them, but I dread having them see Mike. He is so very changed from when they saw him just a little more than a year ago. As much as I write and talk about the changes in Mike, there is no real way to prepare others for the reality of today's Mike.

EMERGENCIES—IT DOES TAKE A VILLAGE
2011

2011. During my nomadic period I made a two-week trip to Southern California, stopping first in the Arcadia/Pasadena area for overnights with longtime friends. From there I drove to Buena Park, headquarters of Morning Glory Press, where I spent a few days with my publisher/friend, then farther south to San Clemente for a visit with friends, then to San Diego, for an overnight with a cousin on my mother's side. From San Diego I drove to Palm Desert where I spent the night with a near-contemporary cousin—she from my father's side—who'd been my partner in cousinhood growing up. Back to Arcadia/Pasadena, and from there I set out to Santa Barbara, the last leg of my trip.

I'd been in daily contact with Rachel during this time, and also in contact with the people who visited Mike regularly. Things were going smoothly in my absence. As for me, it had been good to visit longtime friends. We laughed and cried as we reminisced about Mike. We caught up on each other's lives and families. We ate well, drank well (but not too well), went for walks, shared book recommendations and movie recommendations, stewed about the growing vitriol that seemed to be the new standard for political discourse, and reminisced some more. There were times when I felt almost lighthearted.

I was close to Santa Barbara where I'd planned to spend two nights with Karen, a fellow writer and friend, when my cell phone rang with the distinctive ringtone I'd assigned to Rachel. As soon as safety allowed, I pulled to the side of the road and returned her call. She said Mike was ill and needed to see his doctor. He'd been running a fever all day and was very shaky and unsteady on his feet. If I could get him to the doctor's office by 4 o'clock, they would see him. It was then 3:10, and I was at least five hours from home. Even if I'd been home, I couldn't have made it out to Cameron Park and back to Dr. O's office with Mike before 4. Neither could Dale, Marg, or any of my other local emergency contacts.

"That's unfortunate that no one can take him, because Dr. O'Connor is going out of town on Monday," Rachel said, sounding a bit peeved.

"I'm sorry," I said, "but it is simply physically impossible for me or anyone else I knew to pick Mike up and drive him to the Med Center for a 4 o'clock appointment." I could also have sounded a bit peeved asking why she'd waited so long to call, but I knew when silence was my friend.

The next call came around 6 o'clock, as I was sipping wine and taking in the glorious view of the Santa Barbara bay from Karen's deck. Rachel said we should get Mike to a nearby Rapid Care facility to try to figure out what was going on and to get an order for Tylenol, maybe also an antibiotic.

Although I felt guilty about calling Dale and Marg from my scenic paradise, I didn't know what else to do. They dropped what they were doing, drove to Cameron Park, and took Mike to Rapid Care. When I talked with them later that night, they said Mike had been so shaky and unsteady on his feet, it had taken both of them to get him to the car. He was even more blank than usual and looked lost and confused. Rapid Care did a urinalysis and throat swab, but nothing was conclusive. They got the order for Tylenol and an antibiotic and took Mike back to The Guiding Star.

By the next day, on a Thursday, Mike was a bit better, and I decided to stick with my original plan and stay at Karen's again that night. When I called The Guiding Star on Friday morning, Mike was again running a fever, his neck was swollen, he was eating very little and staying in bed. I headed home.

During my Saturday morning visit, Mike was quite groggy. He sat on the edge of the bed for a few minutes, then lay back down. He made no move to follow me out when I left. Rachel and I talked about another trip to Rapid Care, then followed her inclination to give it another day.

By Sunday morning, Mike's mouth and lower jaw were swollen, and he had blisters inside his lower lip and tongue. I needed to get him to Rapid Care.

It takes two people to manage Mike's getting in and out of the car. Then there's the parking problem. As soon as the driver stops the car in a parking space, or wherever, Mike hurries out and starts walking at a very fast pace to some unknown destination. The driver can't possibly get out and around the car fast enough to get him. So someone always has to be in the back seat, directly behind Mike, to catch him and guide him in the right direction.

I called Dale to ask for transport help, cutting short his happy ramblings through the Sunday Farmers' Market. The same receptionist and aide who'd seen Mike Wednesday night welcomed him back. Cameron Park Rapid Care has to be one of the most user-friendly emergency places in the whole nation.

It turned out that Mike had thrush, a form of yeast infection. The doctor's first choice was to treat it with lozenges, but there was no way Mike would keep a lozenge in his mouth long enough for it to dissolve. We got a prescription for some kind of anti-fungal pills and got him started in the hope that we would see some improvement by bedtime.

Poor Mike. He couldn't say how he was feeling. If asked he'd say "fine." He answered yes or no to other questions, but the answers were not reliable.

"Are you feeling okay?" Yes. "Are you in any pain?" Yes.

We have an appointment with the regular doc on Wednesday. Marg will go with me.

The need for a later visit to Rapid Care occurred on one of Joe and Kathy's visits. While they were walking outside with him, he fell and hit his head on a low brick wall. There was, as always with head wounds, a fair amount of blood, and he was rushed to Rapid Care, this time by ambulance. I arrived at the hospital shortly after he was admitted. Kathy was in the examining room with him, entertaining him as best she could.

Mike remained conscious, needed no stitches, and was released within an hour. I called The Guiding Star to say we would be back within the next 15 to 20 minutes, and asked that someone be watching for us at the door so they could grab Mike when I stopped opposite the entrance.

Once there, I left Mike at "his" dining room table with the understanding that someone would check on him every hour, watching for signs of a concussion. Both the emergency room doctor and Rachel thought a concussion was highly unlikely but, as my mother would have said, it's better to be safe than sorry.

NO MORE NOMADING

July 2011

Sometime around April or May, I renewed my search for a more permanent place to live. I again looked at "affordable housing" possibilities. Most used the same financial criteria for acceptance as had Vintage Woods Senior Apartments. One complex, however, Broadway Senior Center, took medical expenses into consideration, and categorized Mike's residential care costs as "medical." There were 119 one- and two-bedroom duplex units, on well-maintained, nicely land-scaped grounds, with a pool, clubhouse, and laundry facilities—walking distance to markets and cafes, and just blocks from Dale and Marg's. At $500 a month including utilities, it seemed a perfect match. My application was accepted, but at number 38 on the waiting list it seemed unlikely that a place would become available during my lifetime. According to the new director the list hadn't been culled for at least a year, maybe two, so the wait might not be so long.

"Things change fast," she said. "Keep in touch."

Within a matter of weeks I moved from 38 on the list to No. 1. As with Vintage Woods, I pictured myself enjoying time in the Broadway Center pool, sauntering up to Starbucks for a latte, occasionally dropping by Dale's alley garden on my morning walk with Sunny.

When the director called to say two units had opened up, I rushed over, prepared to leave a deposit. I went through both units, one a two-bedroom, the other a one-bedroom. The rooms were quite small, without much natural light. Closet and cupboard space was limited. I doubted that any of my stored furniture would fit. But the outside area and clubhouse were inviting, the location was per-fect, and the price was right. With a single bed, it looked as if the bedroom could hold a small bedside table and chest of drawers. I thought the second bedroom could, with a little maneuvering, serve as my office. There would be room for a small computer table, a bookshelf and two basic file cabinets. I reached for my checkbook, saying I'd like to leave a deposit for the two-bedroom unit.

"Why the two-bedroom?" the director asked.

"I'm a writer. I need some office space."

"A writer?" she said, brightening.

As is often happens when people learn that I write, she told me of a book *she* wanted to write—if only she could find the time. I recommended a couple of "you-can-find-the-time" motivational books for her, then got back to business.

"Do you need first month's for a deposit?" I asked.

Yes, she did, but it would have to be for the one-bedroom. They didn't rent two-bedrooms to singles. It was a hard and fast rule. I went through the one-bedroom again, then asked the director if she would hold it for me for 24 hours, while I mulled things over.

I know. Beggars can't be choosers. And the one-bedroom was certainly larger than the car that was, of sorts, a home base. Still, I was pretty sure that such a cramped space would not be conducive to writing. Of course, I could always go to a coffee place, or library, or some other public space, but even though the book/workshop business had greatly diminished, I still needed a few files. I needed a few books. I thought back to the '40s and to my Granny's trailer—the table with two benches that provided seating for four relatively slim diners, which converted to a bed that could accommodate two very slim sleepers. Maybe I could use such a set-up in the tiny bedroom? I would probably never find another place for only $500 a month. The nearly $200,000 cushion we'd had in 2008 had quickly shrunk to around $30,000. My recent rent-free months had enabled me to stop hemorrhaging money. I didn't want to start again. But as much as I wanted the Broadway Senior Center to work for me, whenever I tried to envision myself in the tiny space, I found myself breathing more deeply, unconsciously fighting a sense of things closing in on me.

I let it go.

I watched the ads, checked Craigslist, drove around, looked at a few advertised places, gradually getting a sense of what was available, where, and for how much. I saw two, 1930s two-bedroom places for $750. Each had spacious rooms with gleaming hardwood floors. The downside was that, although they were in different parts of town, their locations were in competition for the highest crime rates in the Sacramento region. I looked at other rentals that listed for between $700 and $800. Most were shabby, or in high crime areas, or in some noisy, industrial setting. The ones I thought might work weren't interested in renting to anyone with a recent history of bankruptcy.

Dale, in his wanderings about town, had noticed vacancy signs at two large apartment complexes near Sac State. He took a detour and visited both of the places, talking with each of the managers and soaking up details. He later called, identifying himself as my personal shopper, and urged me to take a look at The Reserve on Cadillac Drive. The manager there had assured him that recent bankruptcy need not be a deal breaker.

The apartment was freshly painted, the carpeted areas newly cleaned and in good condition. There was a fenced patio that could be accessed either through living room sliders or an outside gate. It would be nice to be able to open the slider for Sunny first thing in the mornings, rather than having to rush out for a walk while still barely awake. Both bedrooms looked absolutely spacious in comparison to the Broadway place. There was a small kitchen with a dining space that could accommodate up to six people—again if all of these people were of average or less bulk. According to the manager, Marlene, the residents of the 60-unit complex were split about 50/50 between Sac State students and retirees, with a few working couples scattered in. It was quiet.

In July 2010, I signed a one-year lease, got the basics from storage, and moved in, setting up solo housekeeping for the first time in my life. Not exactly solo. Sunny was with me, but there were no human cohabitants.

After taking the $3,200 each month for Mike's care from our teacher's retirement and Social Security income, I was left with about $2,000. My rent would be $950 a month. Tight, but I hoped not impossible. I borrowed enough money against a paid-up insurance policy to cover the deposit and moving expenses and took the leap.

Mike always had very definite ideas about home decor and so did I. He loved antiques and busyness. Royal Doulton figurines and gold-trimmed crystal dishes. Given full reign, he would have filled every inch of space on any table or shelf in our house with a little dish, or silver ornament, a candle in an ornate holder, something he'd brought back from the Soviet Union, or Israel, or from any other number of places he'd visited on choir tours. I loved uncluttered simplicity. We'd lived in a constant state of mostly genial compromise. How far might I take my desire for simplicity when the necessity of compromise was lifted?

Everything needed to be reinvented. Having so long shared the order of my days with Mike, what order would my solo days take? Now I could read all night and sleep all day if I wanted to. Would I? I'd never particularly liked coffee, but I'd liked the companionship and ritual of sharing a cup with Mike each morning while we exchanged sections of *The Sacramento Bee*. We'd had other casual rituals, too. There was the glass of wine before dinner every evening. The after-church Sunday lunches. Would I develop a habit of solo morning coffee? Would I still have a glass of wine in the evenings? What new rituals might I develop?

From the storage unit I took the furniture that would fit the apartment, and the rest went to consignment. shop, Between what I took for the apartment, had already given to Matt and Leesa and to Cindi, or sold through Craigslist or donated to the Goodwill and The Salvation Army, there was not much more left to deal with.

The figurines, fancy vases, little decorative boxes, crystal candle holders and carafes, were either safely packed away in Joe and Kathy's barn, or sitting on consignment in an antique shop in Fair Oaks. Winter clothes were stuffed into my office closet. The storage unit was emptied.

As for rituals, it turned out I did still like a cup of coffee in the morning while I read the newspaper. In the evening, Sunny and I generally sat on the patio around 6 while I sipped wine and she sniffed every inch of ground, as if during her two-hour absence some unwanted critter had infringed on her space.

There was the new ritual of hauling my week's dirty clothes and linens to the laundry room on Tuesday mornings. Tuesdays, because the machines were often taken on weekends and Mondays, and I preferred to have the place mostly to myself. There was the ritual of walking the rent check up to the office every month. Just after coffee and the newspaper, there was the ritual of checking email and sitting at my second bedroom office computer for my daily wrestle with words.

Still, Mike's present state of being was absolutely heartbreaking, and things could only get worse. But he was in a clean, well-managed, stable environment, and although I was thinking of him, sad for him, worried about him every hour of every day, I no longer felt the burden of the day-in, day-out physical care that his condition had required. My financial situation was dismal, but at least the ordeal of bankruptcy was over.

Jerry and Mike had always exchanged cards, sometimes letters, for birthdays and Christmas, and occasionally spoke on the phone. Jerry continued the practice of cards and letters, even after those communications no longer seemed meaningful to Mike. Although Jerry had reached a stage where he hated travel, he made the trip from Florida to visit Mike shortly after the move to The Guiding Star. He was distraught over Mike's worsening condition and, in letters, emails and phone calls, he often expressed his frustration over not being on hand to help out. "If there's ever anything I can do ... " was how he ended every communication. After years of expressing his frustration at not being able to help, of expressing his sincere desire to help, I wrote a letter to Jerry and Jackie, saying that what I most needed at that time was financial help. I said that Jerry had been an amazingly loyal and steadfast brother, and that would remain true whether or not he could offer any kind of financial aid. I said I was writing rather than calling so he and Jackie could talk things over. I didn't want to put him on the spot. The day he received the letter, he called, asking if $400 a month would help. Of course, it would. Perhaps this is just a rationalization on my part, but I think the contribution of $400 a month was also helpful to Jerry, in that he was providing specific, ongoing help for his brother.

A few weeks into my time at the Cadillac Reserve, having taken Sunny for her morning walk along the levee, put the breakfast dishes into the dishwasher, perused and answered email, I sat at my desk, mindlessly gazing out the window, barely noticing the grass-lined, winding pathway that separated my group of apartments from the apartments across from mine. I turned to the tasks at hand—a blog entry that needed editing, a letter of response regarding an inquiry for a school visit, a phone call to Medi-Cal. In the afternoon I would join two friends for a $20 reflexology session. I was slowly finding a life.

ON THE VERGE
OF EVICTION

July 2011 through February 2012

It was a year of ups and downs. Mike wore that now familiar blankness with some random spark occasionally pushing through. He was gradually needing more help with things. He was more frequently incontinent. He sometimes needed help getting dressed. He needed more supervision for showers. Each of these changes added points to the standard residential care assessment chart. More points meant higher fees. If Mike were at any other comparable facility, we would be paying at least $1,000 more. Rachel sometimes mentioned that the administrator had talked with her about bringing our monthly payment in line with the Porto Sicuro fee assessment practices. I was already in the red every month as it was, gradually draining the last of our IRAs. Rachel knew of my financial challenges and, although the possibility of a fee increase was sometimes mentioned, it didn't happen.

Would long-term care insurance have helped? Some. Would veteran's benefits have helped? A lot, but neither of us were veterans. Would money have been easier if we'd not both opted for early retirements? Yes. How about if the economy had not tanked? How about if we'd never used credit cards? These and a truckload of other questions occasionally flitted through my mind, but they didn't linger. The task at hand gave more than enough fuel for thought— to accept the things I could not change, etc., etc.

Even though Mike needed more assistance than he had when he first moved into The Guiding Star, he had calmed down considerably. There were still occasional outbursts, but they were short-lived and less frequent than earlier on. A few of the caregivers took a special interest in him and seemed to genuinely like him. One in particular, Scott, went out of his way to learn about Mike's earlier life. He asked about Mike's previous interests and brought in specific pictures, books and DVDs in hopes of engaging him.

Scott once asked me if Mike liked birds. I told him of the two parakeets,

Bass and Treble, he'd kept in the choir room at SGHS. They'd been a gift from a parent and became choir mascots. Mike was good at delegating work, so along with having a student in charge of taking role, organizing music, and keeping track of robes, someone was always in charge of feeding and cleaning up after the parakeets.

"I could bring in a parakeet!" Scott said. "Would it be okay with you if I brought a parakeet in for him? I've got a cage and everything."

I allowed as how Mike might like that and encouraged Scott to give it a try. He seemed very pleased with the possibility, but after Mike's room had remained birdless for several weeks, I asked Scott if he still planned on bringing one in.

He shrugged. "Regulations," he said.

"Well, nice try. I appreciate that you care, and that you're paying attention."

"I love Mike," he said. He turned to Mike. "We're buddies, right, Mike?"

Mike nodded his head and gave Scott a big smile.

There were other caregivers who connected easily with Mike, one in particular who was pregnant. Mike loved babies. If a friend or fellow singer was pregnant, Mike always wanted to know how she was feeling, when she was due, if she knew whether the baby was a boy or girl. Such questions were beyond him by the time he got to The Guiding Star, but I thought his cooperation with that one caregiver may have had to do with her pregnancy.

Over time I saw a little less of Rachel. That was as it should be. Early on in her role as memory care director, Rachel stayed in one of the Porto Sicuro apartments just a block or so across the driveway from The Guiding Star section. She slept with a walkie-talkie on a table beside her bed, making herself available 24/7.

"I can't rest until I've totally reinvented this place," she once told me.

There was that, being new on the job and wanting to make big changes. The other reason for her apartment stay was that she'd been in a nasty accident with her Sterling convertible, and the car not only needed body work, it needed a new engine. She was waiting for a friend to find and install a rebuilt engine. She and the wrecked car were ensconced at Porto Sicuro for months, but finally the car was fixed, the staff had all been hired and trained by Rachel, and she moved back to her own place in Sacramento. Although I no longer saw Rachel every time I visited, we remained in close email contact.

It was my custom to check Mike's room whenever I visited, see that he had clean clothes, switch from summer shirts and pants according to seasons, and to return whatever purloined books, cards and pictures he'd added to the stack of things he routinely schlepped around.

On one visit, probably in the spring of 2012, Mike's bathroom was filthy. Ten or more dirty cups were on the sink, the basin was grungy, and the floor was sticky with urine. Rachel was not in her office, so I complained to the housekeeping supervisor. She was apologetic but said Mike sometimes lashed out at the housekeepers. They were afraid of Mike and didn't like to go into his room.

"He's not always in his room."

"Well, no, but he's often in there in the mornings when they clean," she said.

"The condition of his room is downright nasty. It certainly wouldn't pass any kind of official inspection," I pointed out.

"I'll get someone down there."

I emailed Rachel about the situation.

"Not acceptable," she wrote back. "I'm on it."

The next time I visited, Mike's bathroom was spotless.

It was around the first of the year that I registered that it had been longer than usual since I'd seen Rachel. Scott paused a moment, then said, "She has a lot on her plate right now."

The following week I sent an email to tell Rachel of an upcoming doctor's appointment for Mike. It was returned as undeliverable. When her work email came back, I tried the home email address she'd given me shortly after Mike moved in. That also came back.

By mid-January 2012, The Guiding Star had a new director, Kyle, who was friendly and nice. I never learned what happened with Rachel, though my guess was that it had to do with not managing the administrative side of things very well. She was great with patients, but her desk was always piled high with undone paperwork. Or maybe it was simply that Rachel was a rolling stone. Whatever it was, I was sorry to see her go. No matter what her administrative faults may have been, she had been totally dedicated to making things work with Mike.

In a journal entry dated January 31, 2012, I'd written:

Mike was in bed when I arrived yesterday morning. One of the caregivers said they'd tried to get him to have breakfast, but he wanted to stay in his room. He was awake, dressed, and lying in bed. There are two comfortable chairs in Mike's room, but I've never seen him sitting in either of them. When I turn the TV on for him, I sometimes suggest that he might be more comfortable sitting in his chair to watch TV. He always remains in bed.

"Did you have breakfast?" I asked, knowing he hadn't.

"Pancakes," he answered.

Matt had sent a postcard of the Getty Museum, telling of his recent trip to LA. I read it to Mike and showed him the picture. Following Rachel's advice, I'm careful not to ask, "Do you know where that is?" or "Do you remember?" I pointed to the picture on the card. "That looks familiar," I said.

"The Getty," Mike replied.

I happened onto an arts channel with a wide range of presentations and chose a symphonic orchestra performance. I was distracted by checking Mike's bathroom for cleanliness, looking through the closet to be sure he had clean clothes, adjusting the thermostat. When I took my place in the chair beside his bed, the symphony had shifted to a ballet, which was holding Mike's attention. "I wonder what ballet that is?" I asked.

"Swan Lake."

Maybe so, maybe not. Next up was Peggy Lee singing "Why Don't You Do Right?" "I always get her mixed up with Kay Starr," I said.

It's amazing how many tricky but non-threatening ways there are to ask a simple question.

"Peggy Lee," Mike said.

"Oh, yeah. We saw her at The Pasadena Playhouse. They brought her out in a wheelchair, but she could still belt out a song." Mike smiled at that.

He dozed. I took some paperwork—always there's paperwork—to a table in the living room and set about filling in the blanks. After a while, probably not more than five minutes, I saw Mike near the entrance. He'd put his shoes on and was carrying Matt's postcard. He looked in my direction and I waved at him. "Shall we go now, hon?" he asked.

"Sure. Let's have lunch first."

I led Mike to the dining room where they'd started serving lunch. I had a cup of soup with him. Once he'd started on his salad and seemed intent on eating, I assured him I'd see him soon and gave him a quick goodbye kiss. He barely looked up from his *food, but by the time I was pulling away from my parking space at the curb, he was punching the key pad at the entrance, trying to get out. He looked up. I waved. He waved back then watched me leave. He was so dejected. Such a sad sight. He vacillates from knowing almost nothing to being fairly aware. Neither state is easy.*

The day after this journal entry, Kyle, the new director, sent an email telling me that Mike had been extremely agitated, violent and aggressive after I'd left. He'd sworn at Kyle, then punched him in the arm several times.

He set a meeting time to "discuss how we move forward in Mike's best interest." Stanley, the facility administrator, would be joining us. I was relieved that Marg was available to go with me to the dreaded meeting. Both her personal and "nursely" insights are invaluable, and her own brand of backup eases the way. I was afraid we were going to hear that they could no longer manage Mike and that we'd have to find another place for him. I dreaded the prospect of moving him, though I knew it might be just around the corner.

Marg and I sat in the office listening to Kyle and Stanley's account of Mike's most recent behavior. They expanded on what I already knew from Kyle's previous email. Tuesday afternoon (the day of my most recent visit) Mike had punched Kyle in the arm several times, fought with a resident, and kicked Mrs. Fitzgerald's dog. All these actions were accompanied by shouts of "No!" and "Fuck!" and "Fuck you!"

They reviewed Mike's care needs. When he entered The Guiding Star just slightly over a year ago, he was at their designated Level 2, which even then was giving him the benefit of the doubt regarding how much he could/would do for himself. He now needed help bathing and dressing. His increased incontinence, coupled with occasional bouts of diarrhea required more housekeeping and hygiene services.

I couldn't quarrel with their assessment, but an increase in fees added urgency to completing the Medi-Cal application process. On the advice of the elder attorney, I'd been working toward getting Mike approved for Medi-Cal coverage, spending hours on multiple phone calls trying to reach the appropriate case worker, getting an "original" Social Security card for Mike to include with the application, getting official notices of yearly benefits from CalSTRS and from Social Security, making copies of last year's state and federal income tax returns, etc., etc. Medi-Cal offered no advantage over our regular Blue Shield insurance plan except that, under some rare circumstances, it would pay for residential memory care—another slim thread of hope.

After meeting with Kyle and Stanley, Marg and I went to Mike's room. He was in bed but got up and followed us to "his" table in the dining room. I showed him the valentines I'd brought for him to sign for the grandkids. Until two years ago, Mike never missed sending them all valentines. One at a time I told him who each card was for and gave it to him to sign. He smiled at the mention of each name and wrote something, sort of, on each card. Mostly what he wrote was illegible. But it was a pleasant activity, and I thought that maybe I should always bring cards for him to sign. I later added my own notes to the valentines and sent the cards on their way.

We took Mike to the patio where Marg managed to help him clip his fingernails. When that task was finished, we followed Mike back inside. He took a seat in the living room where other residents were involved with Wii golfing. We each kissed him and told him goodbye, but he didn't take notice of our leaving. Although that indicated less alertness, it was easier than having him trying to leave with us, or standing sadly at the door as we drove away.

February 2016

Dear Mike,

When was it? Late 2008? Early 2009? It was before your FTD diagnosis, but well into your growing loss of executive function. I was still hoping that a change in meds might bring some improvement, and I suspected that Dr. Carlson was taking a scatter-shot approach to prescribing various drugs. Not that she was negligent or uncaring, but psychotropic drugs were not her area of expertise. Dr. Bertoli helped me get you set up with Dr. Hess, a psychiatrist whom she held in high esteem. He was officially not taking on any new patients, but as a favor to Dr. Bertoli, agreed to see you three or four times—however long it took to evaluate your meds. I drove you to the first visit and spent the hour reading in the waiting room. You came out with a new prescription and careful written instructions on how to start the new med gradually while also gradually cutting back on the old.

You saw Dr. Hess every two weeks or so during this period. Unlike the reputed practices of many psychiatrists, Dr. Hess was not simply a pill dispenser. On our way home from those visits you would tell me of your talks with him. It sounded as if you were telling him the same stories you'd taken to telling everyone, repeatedly, over the past few years—details of your baptism, your mother's craziness, your molestation by an older man who ran a dance school, etc., etc.

At one point, a month or so into your connection with Dr. Hess, you interpreted instructions for a new med to mean you were to take it twice daily. I was sure the instructions indicated a dose of only once a day. A call to Dr. Hess's office clarified that the dosage was indeed meant to be taken once a day. I asked to sit in with you at the next session, to which both you and Dr. Hess agreed. I began seeing Dr. Hess regularly with you, asking the questions I knew you were unlikely to ask, or, if you did ask, to remember the answers.

Eventually, as you became less and less able to follow a conversation, or to provide any accurate information, or to stay in one place for any length of time, I stopped taking you to Dr. Hess and began seeing him on my own. Our conversations centered on you and your condition, and also on how I was managing both practically and emotionally. Now, six years later, I continue seeing Dr. Hess. During the worst of our times, I saw him every week or two. The intent listening he offered, coupled with ques-

tions that led me to a deeper reflection, somehow strengthened me for whatever next step I was facing. It was good to talk with someone who could be an objective listener.

These days I only see Dr. Hess every four to six weeks, but even though my life is much more stable now than it was a few years back, I still find our sessions to be beneficial to my overall emotional health. Other than Dale, for whom I am ever grateful, there are no men in my life that I can share any in-depth, soul-bearing conversation with. Although as a professional, Dr. Hess doesn't exactly qualify as a friend, our conversations get beyond the level of chit-chat. I appreciate that.

All of this was a too-long introduction to what I really wanted to tell you, which is of a recent experience in Dr. Hess's waiting room. The music was calm and melodic, offering a nearly unnoticed backdrop to my attempts to recall details of a puzzling dream I wanted to relate to the doctor. Then came a burst of choral music, the tenor voices so powerful and clean, that I was struck by an image of you, in your tuxedo, on the risers, singing with the Master Chorale. I thought I had put to rest the longing for the you that used to be, but I was suddenly filled with such a great emptiness—so immediate and piercing that it nearly took my breath away. What is it the British say? Gobsmacked?

Would it comfort you to know that you're still such a powerful force in my life?

I expect you always will be. Now that my grief and emptiness is much less constant than before, I've decided to welcome these random gobsmacking experiences, these reminders of you, of us, of love.

Marilyn

ARRESTED!

February 2012

On the way to the parking lot, I check my cell phone, silenced for the past two hours for the sake of movie-goers around me. Two calls—one from The Guiding Star at Porto Sicuro, one from Dale, who is the Guiding Star backup when they can't reach me. In the car I switch to a Bluetooth connection and call Guiding Star. I'm immediately transferred to Stanley.

"We've had a hard time with Mike today,"

"The usual?"

"More than usual. Chuck [one of the caregivers] asked Mike if he wanted orange juice and Mike pushed him to the ground," Stanley said, talking so fast that if the gist of the story were not so familiar it would have been hard to follow. "He yelled, 'Fuck you' at Mrs. Samson—poor, sweet Mrs. Samson who broke into tears and got onto a crying jag that lasted for more than an hour. When I tried to lead Mike back toward his room, he kicked me so hard it drew blood through my jeans. He shoved Mr. Percy. We can't have that."

While I picture the chaos, Stanley pauses for a breath. "We had to call the sheriff," Stanley says. "Mike's been arrested. They took him to Marshall Emergency."

"When?"

"About an hour ago. We had to. We couldn't reach you."

The exit for home dissolves behind me in the rearview mirror as I set my sights on Marshall Hospital.

"You're going to have to find another place for Mike," Stanley says. "We just can't do it any longer. It's not fair to the other residents."

"I know."

"I'm sorry. We've tried everything."

"I know."

Silently thanking the goddess for Bluetooth, I call Dale.

"You talked to The Guiding Star?"

"Yes. I'm on my way to Marshall."

"We're in Tahoe," he reminds me.

"I know. There's nothing anyone else can do anyway."

"Well, but it would be best if you could have company."

"I'm okay."

"Yes, well, other than that, Mrs. Lincoln, how was the movie?"

A sheriff is seated at the door, outside the room where Mike is being held.

"Mrs. Reynolds?" he asks.

I nod and walk into the room. Mike's wrists and ankles are shackled to the bed with hefty iron cuffs. He is heavily sedated but awake. I stroke his bruised cheek, his bruised arm.

"You're in a mess," I say.

Mike smiles, gives a slight nod of his head and closes his eyes. The wreckage left from who he once was haunts me more sometimes than others, but what a sight this is, this remnant of Mr. Fun, charades genius, golden throat, silver tongue, gentle listener, pie baker, and so much more, arms and legs spread, shackled to the corners of the iron bed.

The sheriff peeks in the door and gestures for me to come out.

"It took three of us," he says. "He's strong. There was no reasoning with him."

"He's beyond reason," I say.

The sheriff nods.

"We can 5150 him, put a 72-hour hold on him while he's evaluated, then get him transferred to a more appropriate setting."

I mull it over. If we did this, Medicare would, for a while, pick up the bill. Medi-Cal would take over after that. What a huge financial relief that would be. I glance in at my groggy, shackled, shell of a husband. I can't do it. I can't go the 5150 route. I've seen those "more appropriate" settings. Overworked staff, zombies in hallways, unending cries of distress—"Help!" "Help!" or "Mommy! Mommy!" emanating from six-bed rooms, wafts of odors that insult the olfactory nerves.

"I don't want to 5150 him," I tell the sheriff.

"He's dangerous."

The nurse comes down the hall to say Social Services returned her call. The answer to what resources they might offer was that since Mike's condition was "organic" and not "psychotic," his case is beyond their concern.

I call Stanley and ask if I can bring Mike back for just a few days, until we can find a better placement.

"Four days max," Stanley says.

"Okay."

"We'll have him arrested again if he lashes out."

"I understand."

"You know Mrs. Fitzgerald?"

"The one with the poodle?"

"Yes, the poodle that Mike kicked. In the middle of all of the chaos her heartbeat shot up. She was having palpitations. She has a weak heart as it is. We had to call the ambulance. She's now under observation in the hospital."

Poor Mrs. Fitzgerald, poor poodle, poor Mr. Percy, poor Mrs. Samson, poor Stanley, poor me, poor Mike. Poor gentle Mike. How he would hate who he's become.

I arrange to have someone waiting at The Guiding Star door so they can help me get drugged-up Mike out of the car and into his room.

The sheriff reminds me of how violent Mike's been, how it took three strong men to get him into the squad car just hours ago. He encourages me to reconsider the 5150 alternative.

"I can't bring myself to do that," I tell him.

He shakes his head. I assure him that I'll be okay, that someone will be waiting to meet us at The Guiding Star. Unconvinced, he says he'll follow close behind me on the way back. If I need help, if Mike starts acting up, I'm to blink my lights twice and pull to the side of the road.

I sign the release papers. The sheriff unshackles Mike, and he and an aide get him into a waiting wheelchair. Because Mike is so heavily sedated, it's a struggle to get him into the car and buckled up. True to his word, the sheriff follows close behind me from Placerville to Cameron Park. Seconds after I pull up in front, two aides, one pushing a wheelchair, are out the door. The sheriff, too, comes over to the passenger side of the car to help get Mike out and into the wheelchair. Mike's not uncooperative, just unwieldy.

With Mike safely in the wheelchair, I thank the sheriff and turn to follow the aides as they wheel Mike back to his room.

"Good luck to you," the sheriff says.

"Thank you."

I know I'm going to need more than luck, but I appreciate his kindness.

AFTER THE
GUIDING STAR

February 2012

From my first, tentative explorations of a move to a retirement community, through other explorations of what might be the next move for Mike, Carol Kinsel of Senior Care Solutions had been a major source of information, insight, and support. The morning after Mike's arrest I called to see if she knew of other possibilities. She said there was one private facility in Sacramento that was quite successful in dealing with difficult-to-manage dementia patients. The woman who ran it was a neurologist. It was a top-of-the-line facility, with top-of-the-line $9,000-a-month fees to match. Not possible.

Carol also knew of two local nursing facilities that might possibly take Mike. Another possibility was Sister Sarah's Care Home, a six-bed residential care facility. Carol said the owner and director, Sang Phan, was rather unconventional but had been effective in managing people with extreme behavioral difficulties. Sister Sarah's had an opening, but it probably wouldn't last long. There was also a nursing home/assisted living place an hour away in Fairfield that, except for the distance, sounded as if it might be a good fit.

Dale and I visited both of the nursing facilities Carol had suggested. The first one, a depressingly institutional 80-bed facility, said they weren't equipped to deal with the behavioral difficulties Mike was likely to present. The second one, North Point, was also institutional but with an impressively cheerful and connected staff.

The North Point buildings were clean but, in some sections, bordering on shabby. However, there were three spacious, well-maintained, outdoor areas that residents could access by simply walking through an unlocked door. Mike might do better with more outdoor space in which to wander, but how would he do in a five-bed room? Hard to imagine.

I would much rather see Mike in a more home-like setting than in a 100-plus bed facility. On the other hand, the nursing facility had the available resources of RNs, staff doctors, a psychiatrist, social workers, and a dentist, and it was equipped to deal with all manner of difficulties. Another North Point advantage was that the fee would be at least partially covered by Medicare. After Medicare, Medi-Cal would kick in for approved Medi-Cal patients. There were still more Medi-Cal hoops through which to jump, but, according to a case worker, it looked as if Mike would be approved. What a huge relief it would if the whole financial burden weren't resting on me.

The same day we visited the nursing facilities, I visited Sister Sarah's Care Home, a private residence on about an acre of land in Orangevale, about 18 miles northeast of Sacramento. Sister Sarah (aka Sang), in sweat pants and a T-shirt, met me with a strong handshake and a big smile.

One man and three women were eating lunch at a large table at the end of the kitchen. Sang's husband, Daniel, the facility administrator, was sitting with them. One man was sleeping on the living room couch, half-covered by a fuzzy red blanket. Sang showed me the available room. It was basic but homey. There were two windows in the room, an advantage over Mike's present room, or any room he would have at North Point.

To say that Sang had a bubbly personality would be a gross understatement. She talked the proverbial mile a minute and expressed total confidence that she could deal with Mike. She told me about Ron, the man who was sitting happily at the lunch table. When he first arrived, he might take a bite of food, then throw the rest of it on the floor. He wouldn't talk. If anyone was watching TV, he'd purposely stand in front of it, blocking their view.

"He angel now!" Sang said.

(I don't want to be disrespectful in my attempt to portray Sang's speech patterns. However, if I'd written "He's an angel now," it wouldn't accurately portray Sang.)

Sang showed me the bathroom that Mike would be sharing with Ron and the other man. She took me back to the kitchen where she talked about how she cooked everything from scratch. "Lots of vegetables!" she said. "Even in cookies and cake. Vegetables!"

Ron was still at the table. One of the women was in the living room watching TV. The other was outside, wandering around the enclosed yard.

I followed Sang to the yard, where she pointed out her roses and citrus trees.

The property was fenced around the perimeter with a secure gate. Residents were free to go outside whenever they want to.

"Plenty space!" Sang said. "Everybody need space!"

I told her of Mike's violent outbursts and of his recent arrest.

"Don't worry, honey. He be good here. They all good here."

Daniel joined us outside.

"Right?" she said to him. "They all good here."

Daniel smiled. "Sang has a way. If she tells you your husband will be good here, you can count on it."

"Mike's big—about 6 feet tall, weighs around 180. He's strong."

"Me—not big. Strong!" Sang said. She flexed her bicep. "Feel this!"

I hesitated.

"Come on. Feel this," she said, standing in a body builder pose.

I felt her rock-hard muscle.

"See? No worry!"

On the way home from Sister Sarah's I consider the possibilities. It's $2,800 a month, $200 less than I've been paying, though still a huge stretch. North Point has financial advantages and also a strong support staff. But, for the moment at least, I'm leaning toward Sister Sarah's. Thankfully, Matt will arrive tonight from Walla Walla, and Sharon is coming over early tomorrow. We'll visit North Point and Sister Sarah's in the morning. Dale and Marg will visit Sister Sarah's tomorrow afternoon. Maybe Marg can also see North Point.

In the evening, with the help of martinis, we'll share our observations, pool our opinions and insights, and hope to come up with the best decision for Mike's immediate care. How lucky I am not to be in this alone.

After batting around abstract pros and cons— available resources and support, money, location, rooms, staff, outdoor areas, we try to picture Mike in each of these places. None of us can easily see him in a five-bed room. The constant noise and activity in the North Point hallways would likely raise his level of anxiety to a trigger point. He wouldn't do well with set mealtimes. On the other hand, the North Point staff may have a better chance of finding a balance of meds to counteract his anxiety and explosiveness. And there's the money.

Sister Sarah's? By now we've all, at her insistence, felt her bicep. We've heard her take on food—all fresh, home-cooked, vegetables in everything including desserts. We've been inundated with her good cheer and positive attitude.

"The decor is not exactly to Dad's taste," Matt says.

That's true. The lampshades still sport their cellophane wrap. Furniture is covered with plastic. The place is teeming with plastic flowers. A wallpaper mural depicting a golf course covers one whole wall. Where The Guiding Star was designed and furnished to look like an upscale hotel, Sang's place looks like our Aunt Gladys might have decorated it and, although Mike loved our Aunt Gladys, he did not admire her taste in home furnishings.

"I think Dad's beyond caring about decor," I say. "Even if he's not, my guess is that he'd prefer Sister Sarah's decor to that of North Point."

This turns out to be a two-martini decision, but in the end, the last pretty glass drained, the last stuffed olive eaten, Mike's on his way to Sister Sarah's Care Home.

Both Sharon and Matt offer to help with the cost.

"Not yet," I tell them. "It's not time yet."

After years of graduate school, and more years before Matt landed a tenure track teaching position, plus child care expenses when Leesa worked, and less income when she didn't, Matt and Leesa are barely beyond living month to month. Sharon and Doug are more established financially, but the combined private school tuition for Lena and Subei has got to be a budget strain. There's still a little left in the last of our IRAs.

I tell them the same thing I told Dale after he'd talked with some of the closest 100 Hours friends about possibly pooling resources to help on a monthly basis.

"I'm not totally desperate yet. I'll let you know when I'm totally desperate."

I am grateful beyond words to have such stalwart support. My fervent hope is that I will never become an item in anyone else's budget.

SISTER SARAH'S

February 16, 2012

Moving Mike requires the precision of a synchronized swim team. Knowing how discomfited Mike becomes with any shifting of things, Sharon, Marg and I, go out to The Guiding Star with the purpose of keeping Mike busy and out of his room while Dale and Matt dismantle it. Clothes, shoes, lamps, our bedside table, bedding, CDs, TV, CD player and radio, Mike's stack of snapshots, cards and daybook, 20 or so framed family pictures that hang on the wall of his Guiding Star room—all of that needs to be transferred and set up before Mike enters his new home.

We arrive around 11 to find Mike on the bed in his room. He smiles broadly when he sees us.

"I brought some pictures to show you, Dad," Sharon says. "Do you want to come see them?"

Mike gets up and follows us out to the living room. Sharon shows him pictures of the girls, and old family vacation pictures, many that include him. He gets up and walks toward the hall, in the direction of the room. I lead him back. We take him out on the patio. We tell him stories. We draw him back as he turns to go back inside, as if determined to go back to his room.

"Do you need the bathroom?" I ask.

He nods yes.

I walk him over to the lobby men's room and open the door for him. I wait by the door. He comes out a few minutes later.

"Did you wash your hands?"

He goes back in. Stalling, stalling, stalling is what we're doing. If it's tedious in writing, that's only a hint of the reality.

It's finally close to lunchtime, and the four of us sit at Mike's table. The caregivers know what we're up to and try to help by bringing us snacks and drinks. When it's truly lunchtime and the others are in the dining room, they bring Mike his soup and salad. After a few tastes of soup, Mike gets up. One of us calls his attention to his salad. He sits back down. One bite, then up again.

Finally, after more of this, encouraging him to eat, taking him out on the patio, showing more pictures, and doing it again and again, we hear from Dale. They're at Sister Sarah's. Daniel was there waiting for them when they arrived. The three of them unloaded Dale's truck, and the big stuff is now in Mike's new room. They just need to make up the bed, get pictures on the wall, and clothes in the closet and chest of drawers. He figures they'll be ready for Mike in about 45 minutes. We stall a little longer, then take Mike to the car.

Once in the car, I explain to Mike that we're taking him to a new place. I assure him we want him to be someplace where he will be relaxed and comfortable. I remind him of his recent horrible experience with the sheriff and tell him we wanted to do everything we can to keep that from happening again.

"I'm sure you don't want that to happen again, do you?"

He shakes his head no.

It's impossible to know how much or how little Mike understands, but I must at least try to let him know what's happening.

Marg calls Dale to say we're about 15 minutes away from Sister Sarah's. They want another 45 minutes.

Sharon suggests we stop for a latte. As soon as she says it, we all know how ridiculous that would be. Mike can't stay in one place for more than a minute or two. We're going to take him into a Starbucks?

Maybe a drive-through? But as soon as the car stops, he'll get out. We decide to see more of the sights of Orangevale. When we get to Sang's street, we turn in the opposite direction of the facility. We drive slowly past a small park where some moms are pushing little kids in the swings. We drive slowly past a high school. Slowly around another block. We drive slowly toward Sister Sarah's Care Home. Marg calls Dale to ask that someone be watching for us to buzz us in so we won't have to sit waiting at the gate. That works.

Sang meets us at the front door. "Michael!" She extends her hand to him. "I'm Sang. I'm your new friend."

Mike shakes hands with Sang. "Oh, very good handshake! You very handsome man."

Mike stands smiling, watching Sang.

"Come see your room. Very beautiful!"

Dale and Matt meet us in the entry way. They greet Mike with hugs. Mike follows Sang down the hall to the last door on the right. We follow Mike. The room has a familiar look—same bedspread, family pictures on the wall, Mike's Aunt Ursie's antique lamp. There are still more pictures to hang, but we can do that later. The room already looks like it's Mike's.

After 15 minutes or so, seeing that all is relatively well, Dale and Marg go home. Matt, Sharon and I stay for another couple of hours. We walk outside with Mike; we talk with Sang and Daniel. Ethel, one of the women residents, seems taken with Matt and follows him around for a while. I sit with Mike at the table while he eats a piece of cake.

"Little bit chocolate. Little bit sugar. Lots carrots and zucchini."

Across the table from Mike, Ron is also eating cake.

When he's finished with his cake, Ron turns his attention to me.

"When are you going to kiss me?" he demands to know.

I laugh. "Never," I tell him.

"But I thought we were engaged," he says.

"Nope. See this guy over here?" I say, putting my hand on Mike's shoulder. "He's my husband."

"He's big," Ron says, then leaves the table.

The man who I now know is "John" is asleep on the couch.

"He sleep a lot," Sang says. "Very tired."

Sang says to Mike, "You my friend? We friends, right?"

Mike smiles and nods.

"You handsome guy! You know?" He smiles and nods again.

Matt, Sharon and I leave around 4 in the afternoon. Later we have dinner at the Dodsons'. We start with our traditional pre-dinner martinis, just one apiece tonight. Marg has again done her kitchen magic—baked salmon, tasty garden fare, garlicky mashed potatoes. Dale's made a lemon-blueberry tart, from scratch. The move went more smoothly than any of us dared imagine. We are celebratory. And worried.

After dinner I take a deep breath and call Sang. Mike had eaten dinner and was now in the living room with the others, watching TV. Whew!

The morning after the move, about 5 o'clock, I drive Matt to the airport. Once back home I sit on my hands to keep from calling Sang too early. She'd said mornings were very busy. Best not to call before 10. I walk Sunny, do a little cleaning, and pay a few bills until, finally, the clock says 10.

Sang answers and I, with some apprehension, ask how Mike's doing.

"I give two thumbs up!" she says.

"Really?"

"Yes! He very happy with me! When I help him in shower, I sing 'You Are My Sunshine.' He not sing a single word then, but after he sing with me and Daniel."

"Really?" I ask again, having apparently minimized my vocabulary to one word.

"He have good voice! We record DVD for you."

Sang tells me Mike went to bed around 11 when she and Daniel did, slept all night, got up for breakfast, then went back to bed.

"He know where everything is—his room, the bathroom, everything. He fine, honey! You go get something you like eat. Put your feet up. Read book."

On the afternoon of my next visit, Mike is at the table eating what appears to be a jelly sandwich and drinking a glass of milk.

"Hi, Mike," I say, pulling a chair up next to him.

"Hi, Marilyn," he says, smiling broadly.

At our most recent visit to the doctor, when Dr. O'Connor asked Mike if he knew who those two ladies were who were with him, Mike said, "Marilyn and Marg." But today is the first time he's actually spontaneously said my name during this past year.

Sang joins us at the table and tells me that Mike has had a bit of diarrhea this morning. The jelly slathered on bread is masking something to combat this tendency.

Earlier at breakfast, Ethel tried to talk to Mike. Sang could see that Mike was getting irritated, so she found something on the other side of the room to interest Ethel. "I read body language," she says.

Daniel shows me the video he took yesterday evening—Mike and Sang singing "You Are My Sunshine," and another bit of Mike and Sang dancing. Mostly Sang was the one dancing, but Mike was smiling.

As I pull into Sister Sarah's driveway one day the following week, I'm surprised to find Mike sitting behind the wheel of Daniel's truck, parked in the driveway. I open the door on the driver's side.

"Going somewhere?" I ask.

"No." Mike says, keeping his hands on the steering wheel and gazing out the windshield as if watching for traffic. I leave Mike in the truck and go inside to talk with Sang.

"Mike's in the driver's seat of Daniel's truck," I tell her.

"That okay. No keys."

She catches me up on how things have been going. She says that instead of trying to get residents to conform to any particular schedule, she watches to see what develops naturally. She says Mike's developing a pattern. He generally gets up around 7, has a cup of tea or something light, then goes back to bed until 10 or 11. Then he has more to eat and is up for the rest of the day. In the afternoon Sang may keep Mike's door locked for a while to encourage him to be out and about with the rest of the them.

I've brought another pair of pajamas for Mike, and as I carry them toward his room, Sang follows.

"Don't worry—his bed not made," she says, then tells me that if things seem to be becoming tense between Mike and another resident, she asks him to come help her, leads him into his room and they make the bed together. By the time they go back to the living room, the mood has changed. Later, she rumples his bed again so it will be ready for the next distraction.

I'm amazed at how well things are going with Mike at Sister Sarah's. Do I think there's going to be trouble ahead? Yes. The very nature of FTD means there is always trouble ahead. But what a sweet respite we're having.

UPS AND DOWNS AT SISTER SARAH'S

February 2012 through September 2013

Sang and Daniel, along with Sang's 17-year-old son, Ronnie, live on the premises. Ronnie has his own basement "apartment," but he takes meals upstairs and in the afternoons is often at the dining room table doing homework. On rare occasions Sang and Daniel hire another caregiver, usually one of Sang's sisters, for a short night out, but that's a rare occurrence. Daniel maintains the building and grounds and is around for backup in the early mornings and evenings. But because he has his own contracting business that specializes in remodeling jobs, some small and some more extensive, he's often on a job during the day. Sang is on the job 24/7. I don't know how she does it. I couldn't, but I'm glad she can.

Daniel laughs when he tells me it's thanks to the recession that he's got a lot more time to help at home. But he says when he's out on a job and it gets close to 5, he's eager to get back. "I want to see what the kids have been up to," he says.

Both Daniel and Sang seem to genuinely like Mike. "We're buddies, aren't we Michael?" Daniel often says, to which Mike usually gives a faint smile and nods his head. Sang says, "Today you a 10, Mr. Mike! I give you two thumbs up!" When one or the other of them put their arms out and ask for a hug, Mike opens his arms to them.

Mike has developed a pattern of walking in a loop, out the front door, around the side of the house, into the back door, through the living room, down the hall, out the front door, etc. etc. I'm glad he's got room to roam here. I no longer have to deal with the pacing caged tiger vision of him that haunted me for so long.

Although the larger, upscale facilities such as The Guiding Star are more appealing to the eye, and tout programs for socialization, physical stimulation, music therapy, a caring specially trained staff, etc., etc., the care Mike received at Guiding Star was not nearly as personal and individualized as at Sister Sarah's. One of the problems at the Guiding Star was that Mike had to deal with different caregivers every day—changing shifts, staff turnover, vacation times, etc. Some of the Guiding Star caregivers knew and liked Mike, and could generally manage him. Others, though, didn't like Mike, were afraid of him, and inept when it came to managing his behavior. At Sister Sarah's it was Sang and Daniel, mostly Sang, all day, every day. It turned out that the smaller setting was a much better set-up for Mike. Really, it was a better set-up for me, too. Unlike the larger place, whenever I called Sister Sarah's to ask about Mike, whoever picked up the phone knew exactly what was going on with him and could give a full report without trying to find his chart.

During his first month at Sang's, Mike didn't hit anyone. Not once. Then one month to the day, he suddenly starts lashing out again. He hits Sang when she's showering him. But, ever cheerful, she tells me, "That okay! No problem, honey! He not hurt me! Just bam, bam, bam, but not hard!"

He hits residents if one or another gets too close to him. That is a problem. Being totally incontinent now, Mike's farther along the assessment scale than when we first moved him in. The new monthly fee is $3,200 plus another $100 for incontinence supplies.

After many months of filling out form after form, and providing copies of last year's income tax return, and waiting for an hour and a half at the Sacramento County Department of Human Assistance to be interviewed by a social worker, and then providing the W-2 forms and income statements from Social Security that had not been requested earlier, and signing an "I Am Not a Liar" paper in the presence of a notary public, finally, Mike is officially approved for Medi-Cal with no share of costs. I'm not sure if that will offer any financial relief or not. It would have had we chosen North Point, but Medi-Cal doesn't typically cover care provided by six-bed residential facilities. I've heard of a pilot waiver program that may cover a few such facilities, but Sister Sarah's Care Home is not part of that program.

A side note here about the Department of Human Assistance. The people who work there are doing a tough job, seeing a steady stream of needy folks all day long, day after day, many of them who've not brought in the right paperwork or haven't understood the forms. One of the Human Assistance workers was polite and treated me with respect, but my general experience was one of being treated with grumpy condescension, as if I were nothing more than a brainless number. If dealing with Human Assistance is a humiliating experience for me, a well-educated native English speaker, how much worse it must be for the Colombians, the Vietnamese, the Mexicans, the Ukrainians.

Given my income after paying for Mike's care, I fell into the poverty category. Maneuvering the Medi-Cal maze I was in gave me added insight and empathy into the lives of the truly impoverished.

Basic lab tests, blood panel and stool sample had not revealed the cause of Mike's ongoing bouts of diarrhea. No matter how Sang worked with Mike's diet, diarrhea had become a near daily occurrence. The ongoing incontinence and chronic diarrhea required a higher level of care than at first anticipated. Sang and Daniel arranged a time to meet with me and talk about about Mike's increased needs. Following the standard assessment criteria, they said, the fee for someone with Mike's needs was around $4,200. They needed to raise their fee to stay in line with that assessment. The new payment would start in six weeks.

"That's a big, sudden jump," I said.

I told them I had absolutely no doubt that their care was worth every penny of that, but I didn't see how I could manage it.

The next time Marg visited, Sang went over the fee assessment with her, how they hadn't factored in Mike's consistent incontinence or chronic diarrhea when we came in at the base rate. Sang showed Marg a picture of a shit-smeared floor where Mike's mess had leaked from his Depends.

"You see? I clean! Every day I clean! It okay! My job! No place else do this for what Marilyn pay."

As a hospice nurse, Marg was familiar with the assessment charts. What Sang was asking was not unreasonable, given the circumstances. Marg told Sang the same thing I had. Their care was certainly worth $4,200 a month, but she knew my financial situation, and I simply would not be able come up with that amount on a monthly basis.

I called Carol Kinsel to get contact information for the Fairfield place. She thought that would probably be the best match for Mike if he couldn't stay at

Sang's. She also suggested we check out St. Anthony's, which was a waiver program facility closer to home than Fairfield. I made appointments at both places and, because the world of memory care and assisted living was a small world, I called Sang to tell her I'd be looking at other places. I wanted that information to come from me, not through the local residential caregivers gossip network. I told her my all-time first choice of a place for Mike was with her, but I couldn't manage $4,200 a month.

Sang was upset. "Nobody take care of Mike like I do!"

"Right. I wish he could stay with you for the duration, but it's just not possible at $4,200 a month."

"I thought you happy with me!"

"I *am* happy with you. It's been so nice to have Mike in a place where people actually like him. I hate the thought of moving him again."

On my next visit Sang asks, "You find better place than here?"

"There is no better place than here! This is the place I want Mike to be, but look, this is how things are for me."

I take the tablet and pencil from the counter. I write down Mike's take-home pay from his CalSTRS retirement, then mine. Mike's net Social Security, then mine. The total comes to $4,370. "At $4,200 I'd be left with $170 a month to live on. How could I manage that?"

"Ron's family pay $4,200 and he not even incontinent!"

Now *I* want to hit her bam, bam, bam!

As Mike walks past the kitchen on his loop Sang says, "You very handsome today! Gimme a thumbs up!"

Mike smiles and sticks up his right thumb. She hands him a quarter of a sandwich from a waiting plate. He takes a bite as he walks out the door.

"He don't sit very long, honey, but no problem. He get plenty food this way."

In truth, except for breakfast when Mike might sit briefly to slurp cereal from a bowl, nearly all of his food intake occurs on the run. That, and whatever he can glean from the two kitchen cupboards that are accessible to him.

By the time I am ready to leave, Mike has had six of those pieces of sandwich. He's eaten two or three. The others he's taken a bite from, then put down on the bookcase, or the table in the entry, or maybe somewhere out in the patio.

"He remember," Sang says. "He come back for it."

As if on cue, Mike picks up the sandwich piece as he passes the bookshelf and pops it into his mouth. He is so much better off here, where Sang has adapted to his preferences, than he would be at a place with set mealtimes and table arrangements. I don't even want to think about moving him, but what can I do?

St. Anthony's was big, with set mealtimes, and they couldn't deal with volatile behavior. The Fairfield place was a possibility, though. Cheerful. Plenty of secure outdoor space. The director, James Franklin, was confident they could work with Mike. They were not on the waiver program, but he said they worked with people according to their budgets.

"He doesn't do well with set mealtimes."

"I don't either," James said, laughing. "We have windows of time for meals, but if someone misses that window, they can always go to the kitchen and get whatever it is they missed."

I liked James. I liked the place. The hour drive each way didn't appeal to me, but I thought Mike might do okay there. I made another appointment with the director for the following week, so Sharon and I could visit together. She, too, liked the director and the facility. There was a vacancy in the memory care unit. The monthly fee would be $2,200. "How high might that rate go if Mike turns out to need more care than he does right now?" I asked.

"That rate will stay the same for the duration of his care," James said. "It will be secured in your contract."

Sharon and I stood talking in the parking lot. We agreed that this could be an option. It would be a hellacious drive during peak traffic hours, but not bad if the timing were right. The monthly fee was much more realistic for me than I was currently paying at Sang's, and a huge contrast to what their increase would be.

Sharon left to pick Subei up from a soccer game. I went back inside and asked James if he could hold the spot for Mike for a few days.

"Sure," he said. "We'll hold it for a week."

I thanked him and drove back home, wondering how it would feel to make this same drive once or twice a week—more often when the inevitable other problems arose.

A few days after our Fairfield visit, Daniel emailed to say he and Sang would like to meet with me again. When I showed up the next afternoon, they told me they'd talked things over. They were dedicated to Mike. They thought he was better off with them than he would be elsewhere. I agreed. They decided they would like to keep Mike at the current rate of $3,200 for the next six months. Daniel said they wanted to see "what good might happen with Mike here. We can re-evaluate at the end of six months."

Even though the Fairfield facility made sense financially, Mike was doing relatively well with Sang and Daniel. Another move would be a crapshoot. Then there was the distance. Relieved, I called James to cancel our hold on the room at Fairfield.

Daniel called Dr. O'Connor regarding Mike's chronic diarrhea and also his volatility. He said they talked at length and that Dr. O'Connor had asked that Sang and Daniel FAX him regularly with details of Mike's daily actions. Perhaps a change of meds was in order.

Trazodone, Depakote, Lipitor, and Zyprexa were among the array of drugs Mike was taking when he moved to Sister Sarah's Care Home. By that time I was not paying as close attention to his drug regimen as I had in the past. As far as I could see, nothing made much difference. An increase in the dosage of Depakote shortly after Mike moved to The Guiding Star might have lessened his outbursts for a while. Zyprexa calmed him for a while. Whatever calming effect such drugs might have, though, were short-lived.

At the top of the list of many of Sang's strongly held opinions was her take on drugs—the fewer, the better. None was best. Most people would probably agree with that in theory, but in practice we generally take the prescribed blood pressure medication to diminish the likelihood of a stroke. Or we resort to medicating our insomnia. Or we take pain meds because of a bad back. Then there are the antidepressants and heart regulators. But unlike most of the rest of us, Sang, was a woman who held fast to her convictions.

On our first visit, before we'd even moved Mike in, Sang had told us how when Ron first came there he slept all of the time. "Even when he wake, he fuzzy. Too fuzzy! No talk!" she said. She went on to say how she'd gradually weaned him off all drugs.

"Look at him now! You look at his bright eyes when you go back out." She was obviously proud of her accomplishment.

Daniel said Ron's family thought Sang was a miracle worker.

After the first few weeks of Mike's stay, Sang had asked, "You trust me?"

"I do trust you," I said. "You're doing a great job with Mike."

"Okay," she said, lowering her voice a few decibels below her usual cheerleader volume. "Little bit. I take little bit, slow, slow, get Mike off too many drugs. Don't tell. Okay?"

I didn't have to think long before I gave her the go-ahead. I'd seen enough of her work with Mike and also with the other residents to see that the wisdom of her instincts and intuition went beyond the usual caregiver approach. Although Sang didn't have the medical or academic background that Rachel had, she was equally keen in her understanding of her charges. Not only that, but Sang was on the job 24/7. Literally 24/7. Marg called Sang "crazy saint." That seemed an apt description.

Sang repeatedly reminded me that this slow reduction of Mike's drugs was to be kept in strictest confidence. Their license could be revoked if her dose-altering practices were to be revealed. They could also have their license revoked for cutting Mike's nails, something that regulations demanded be done either by family or an RN rather than a designated caregiver. Mike was still mostly able to cut his own fingernails, though he sometimes needed help with the nails on his right hand. I gave Sang my full approval to offer help with his fingernails when needed and also to cut Mike's toenails. My approval was nothing when weighed against official regulations, though.

Dr. O'Connor was also of the "less is better" school of drug use. In one of Daniel's fax reports to Dr. O'Connor he'd mentioned a persistent twitching of Mike's right wrist whenever he walked or stood. This had started several months ago when Mike was still at The Guiding Star. The twitching stopped when he used his hand to hold onto a glass or pick up a fork, but when his hand wasn't in action, the twitching resumed. This was possibly related to FTD, but it was also a possible side effect of Depakote.

Interestingly, the possible side effects of Depakote are surprisingly similar to the symptoms of FTD: confusion, trouble sleeping, anxiety, changes in patterns and rhythms of speech, restlessness, problems with memory, etc., etc. Depakote was prescribed as an anti-seizure medication. As with many of the drugs Mike either was or had been on, there seemed to be some difference in his behavior when he had first started taking Depakote, but not much and not for long.

When Dr. O'Connor learned of the hand twitching he decided to cut back on the Depakote dosage. That seemed to make a slight difference, though "slight difference" was hard to quantify.

I don't know how much of this was done on Dr. O'Connor's orders and how much was Sang's personal doing, but within five months of Mike's move to Sister Sarah's, he was down to just one anti-anxiety drug, Seroquel. He was off all of the drugs he'd been on when he left The Guiding Star: Trazodone, Depakote, Celexa and Lipitor.

"Michael brighter now—not foggy," Sang said. "Too many drugs before. Not good."

I didn't see any difference in Mike's brighter/foggy state, but just on general principles I was glad to have him off such a large assortment of powerful pharmaceuticals.

My feeling was that Mike's level of brightness vs. fogginess was generally random, related to the havoc within the chaos of his FTD-afflicted brain. Whatever the cause, nothing was predictable. Usually he greeted me with a quick smile and hug, barely pausing in his counter-clockwise loop through the house, around the yard, and back through the house. Usually he smiled at me when he came through again. At other times he might pause and look at me as if I were a stranger, or he might peer at me, intently, for several seconds, perhaps trying to figure out who I was.

Months into his stay at Sister Sarah's, Mike continued to lash out at residents and they were generally afraid of him. Ron called him "that big guy" and tried to keep his distance. The others, two wheelchair-bound women and the sleeper never crossed Mike's path so they were safe. Well, relatively safe. Mike did slap the hand of one of the women when she held onto a plate of food that he was trying to take from her.

Then there was Helen. She also walked around outside, though not with such a distinct pattern as Mike's. Helen often was outside when I drove in, and she always offered a pleasant greeting as I got out of the car. "Did you bring them with you?" she might ask with a smile, or "Can I have the roses now?" or some other short question that meant nothing to me but something to her. I usually responded, "They may be here later," or "I'm sorry, I forgot the roses." She would nod, as if satisfied with my response, then walk away. But she walked. And Mike walked. And they each assumed they had full right of way no matter where or when. If they both arrived at the front door at the same time, neither gave way. Sang was always on the job, and Daniel was there often, but as alert as they were, Mike and Helen sometimes reached the same place at the same time unnoticed.

I knew from Sang's reports that Mike had on more than one occasion pushed Helen out of his way, and that Helen had, more than once, shouted insults at Mike, but it wasn't until an afternoon in early May that I got to witness the Mike and Helen Show first hand. Mike, on his usual loop, had just passed me in the entryway. Helen opened the front door to come in just as Mike was on his way out.

"No!" he shouted and shoved her aside.

"You goddamned son of a bitch!" she yelled after him.

Without the slightest pause in his trajectory Mike yelled back, "Fuck you!"

By that time, Sang was standing with an arm around Helen's shoulder, calming her as she led her into the kitchen, away from Mike's path. I met Mike as he came through the back door.

"How're you doing?" I asked, moving in beside him and following along.

"Fine!" he said, still sounding angry. He continued to walk toward the front door. I fell behind, giving him full access to the doorway.

With Helen eating a snack at the table, and Mike walking his unobstructed pathway, I returned to the kitchen where Sang was preparing dinner.

"It okay, honey," she said to me, referring to Mike and Helen's altercation. "We make it work. No worry."

By mid-May, Mike had taken to going shirtless. Shortly after Sang dressed him in the mornings, he would take his shirt off. She'd help him put it on again. He'd take it off. He'd also stopped wearing shoes.

At Sang's request I wrote a note for her to keep on file, saying that I understood that Mike often removed articles of clothing repeatedly during the course of any given day, that this was one of many behaviors common to victims of FTD, and that Sang was in no way negligent in attending to Mike's dress. It was important for Sang to have this statement on file for the sake of a drop-in visit from a licensing monitor.

For months I'd been making phone calls and filling out form after form to get Mike approved to enter an Assisted Living Waiver facility, and also getting information on what it would take for Sang and Daniel to become licensed as an ALW facility. My greatest hope was that Sister Sarah's Care Home would soon be ALW-certified, and that Mike's fees there would be covered, or at least partially covered.

The first several months Mike was with Sang and Daniel, he would often sit on the couch for an hour or so and watch TV, but then he became too restless even to do that. So he walked. And walked. Morning, noon and night, he walked. The fairly frequent diarrhea was an ongoing problem. Lashing out at other residents was an ongoing problem.

Although Mike never sat at the table for more than a few minutes, he was eating all of the time. Sang handed him food as he walked past the kitchen. Pieces of sandwiches, pieces of cheese, healthy finger foods. For food that required utensils and a plate, she'd leave a plate of whatever they were having for dinner, plus a fork, on the entryway table and Mike would help himself to a bite as he passed by. Sometimes he'd move the bowl to a bookshelf in the living room, or to a side table by the couch, but he'd always come back to it, seldom leaving any food uneaten. He was eating constantly, but he was also steadily losing weight. When he left The Guiding Star, he weighed about 190, down from the 223 pounds he'd weighed when he first entered. Now with the scales at 181, he was probably at his ideal weight.

The tremor in his right wrist came and went. There were a few puzzling times when Mike leaned to his right at an extreme angle, walking bent and crooked. This might last for a day or two, then he'd straighten up again.

I saw Mike every week, as did Marg. Sharon came when she could, usually at least once a month. Matt managed to get down three or four times a year. Although his visits weren't weekly, Dale was on call as needed. And Dale was a constant backup for me, helping with a myriad of daily tasks, including beautifying my new apartment patio with plants—in the ground, in pots, in hanging baskets. Mine was the most colorful patio in the whole compound.

Through it all Sang was, indeed, a crazy saint. She talked a mile a minute, showed off her muscles, wanted hugs almost as a sort of punctuation. She made Norman Vincent Peale look like a grump. She cooked tasty and healthy meals. The residents were always clean and well-groomed and she kept the house clean. She oozed confidence, never doubting that she knew what was best for her charges and that she could provide them with the best possible care. She often told me that she could keep Mike through to the very end. She could work with hospice. If there came a time when he needed oxygen, or a colostomy, or was wheelchair-bound, she could take care of it all. That was reassuring.

Sharon and Subei planned to visit one Friday about six months into Mike's stay there. It was a school holiday for Subei, but not for Lena. Sharon offered her the choice of going with them to visit Grampa or going to school. Lena, who was then in a thankfully short-lived phase of not liking school, chose Grampa. I hated to have the grandkids see Mike as he was, but I also hated for them not to see him, and for him not to see them. He always lit up when he first saw any of them, and although his pleasure may have lasted only a nanosecond, it did seem to be pure pleasure.

This was the girls' first visit to see Mike since we'd moved him from Porto Sicuro. It was my practice to call ahead when I visited, and on this day Sang met us in the driveway as we got out of the car.

"Beautiful!" she said to Subei. "So beautiful. Give me a hug!" She opened her arms to Subei and Subei complied. "I love you!" Sang told her.

She then turned to Lena. "Beautiful lady! Give me a hug!" Lena held back. "Come on! Hug!" Sang said, walking close with her arms out. Lena gave a half-hearted hug and walked on. Mike came out on his loop and gave a big smile when he saw us. He stood still long enough to get a hug from each of us, then, still smiling, he walked on.

We went inside and met Mike coming back through. Sharon always brought a treat for Mike, and on this day I think it was chocolate chip cookies. He paused in his loop long enough to take a cookie from her outstretched hand, then walked on. Sharon watched with tears streaming down her cheeks.

We watched more loops, heard Sang's report of Mike's behavior, eating habits, and their progress, or not, in dealing with his chronic diarrhea. Helen came in from outside and gave Sang a big, toothless grin.

"Oh, Helen! Not again?" Sang said, half laughing. "Go back and find your teeth. You'll need your teeth for that good cake you like."

When Helen went back outside, Sang said, "She bury her teeth in the yard now. All the time, bury her teeth."

Helen came back inside, empty-handed.

"Come on, Helen. Show me," Sang said, leading Helen back outside.

After a few more loops, a few more offered cookies, we were ready to make good on our promise to Lena of a stop at an In-N-Out Burger. As we stood in the driveway, saying our goodbyes, Sang gave out hugs, telling us she loved us. Lena again held back. Sang again insisted.

"A hug, beautiful lady!"

As we drove away, Lena allowed as how next time she'd stay in school.

"I know," I said. "It's really hard to see Grampa like this."

"It's not Grampa. It's that happy, hugging, Sang woman!"

Sang was, admittedly extreme, but I preferred happy and hugging for Mike to anything I'd seen elsewhere.

GOOD NEWS?
September 2013

After several setbacks in the ALW licensing process, Sang and Daniel finally got all the required items signed off by the licensing agency. There were no big problems with the licensing, just time-consuming tasks that had to be completed before they could be officially designated an Assisted Living Waiver facility. The caregivers, including Sang's sister, her son, and anyone else they might call on for occasional help, all had to be fingerprinted. Even though they'd all had TB tests when Sister Sarah's first opened, they needed to be tested again. The automatic gate opener needed to be upgraded to meet new fire department standards, etc., etc.

It was months after Mike was officially okayed as a potential ALW resident before Sister Sarah's license came through, but what a relief it would be to finally get some financial assistance. It seemed that all was in order, but then, oops, although all of the requirements had been checked off, the man who actually issued the licenses retired, and there was not yet a replacement. Phone calls weren't being answered. It seemed there was no place to turn. Carol Kinsel jumped in to try to move things along, but none of it was easy. I kept hoping, month to month, that there would be a shift.

I was getting closer to rock bottom. The bankruptcy procedures were finished, and I'd come away from that as clear as anyone could from bankruptcy. It stopped the nasty phone calls and letters, but that didn't do anything to ease my ongoing monthly money challenges. It seemed within reason that Mike's residential care expenses might soon be at least partially alleviated through the ALW program or through some aspect of Medi-Cal, but in the meantime I was still paying out more than was coming in month after month after month.

Early one September evening, after being out running errands and grocery shopping, I settled in to get caught up with email and paperwork tasks. There was a message from Daniel to call Sang. "Good news," he wrote, saying I could call as late as 1 in the morning.

I got my hopes up for the good news to be word that Sister Sarah's Care Home had received the official ALW license. I called Sang.

"Good news, honey! I found very good placement for Mr. Mike!"

She went on in her mile-a-minute style. A hundred dollars less each month. The woman running the place had even more experience than Sang did. Sang knew this because they'd worked together a few years back, before either of them had opened their own facilities.

I was stunned and could hardly process the "good" news. Sang had all kinds of justifications, insisting that this would be best for Mike.

After an abundance of miscommunications, what I was left with was that Mike and Helen were becoming more combative with one another and that there was a risk of someone being hurt during one of their tussles.

I was reeling. My confusion and worry soon turned to anger. Whatever happened to "It okay, honey, we make it work. No worry!"? Or to Sang's frequent and seemingly heartfelt assurances that they were dedicated to taking care of Mike through the very end?

After a worried and sleepless night, I emailed Daniel to ask for clarification.

As I sat waiting for a response, still stunned by the news that Mike must leave the place where he'd received such good, enlightened care, I looked back over my email correspondence with Daniel. Over the course of a year, from late March 2012 to early April 2013, there were 48 emails from Daniel. Those were only the ones I'd saved. My guess was that Daniel and I had consistently had email contact three to four times a week. He sometimes sent a video of Sang and Mike "dancing," or photos of Mike outside by the roses.

Emails back and forth had clarified certain details that had been confusing in conversations with Sang. During a visit early on in Mike's stay at Sister Sarah's, Sang and I had a long, one-sided conversation regarding various possibilities for the incontinence supplies I was to provide. On my way home I stopped at Target to buy what was needed, then, still in the parking lot, realized my head was spinning with possibilities. Sang had talked about Depends Adjustables, and briefs, Tena Heavy Protection and Always Discreet. I left Target without going inside, which is usually my natural impulse anyway.

A quick email to Daniel had clarified things—Depends Briefs, M/L, best deal at Costco. Together, mostly through emails, Daniel and I had navigated the tricky details of ALW licensing and placement approval. Sometimes the emails we exchanged were simply book or movie recommendations. My hope on the morning after receiving such questionable "good news" was that Daniel could shed some light on this shocking turn of events.

In response to my "I don't understand. Can you enlighten me?" email, Daniel suggested I come talk to Sang in person. I asked what a good time might be, not wanting to show up for a conversation if there were other visitors. Sometime between 2 o'clock and 4 o'clock was the preferred time that day. At 1:30 I took four supermarket cookies from the stash I kept in the freezer, put them in a baggie, and drove to Orangevale.

On the way to Sister Sarah's I tamped down my anger with reminders of how amazingly good both Sang and Daniel had been with Mike—what excellent care he'd received there over the past year and a half. I reminded myself that they actually enjoyed Mike. They were lighthearted with him. They had been more than fair in establishing a monthly rate for me. I needed to stay open to whatever Sang had to say.

Sang was always a fast talker, but faster still when she was nervous. As Mike looped past me, he reached for a cookie, took a bite, put it on the bookshelf as he walked past, took another bite on his next circle through, left it on the entry table, round and round, cookie after cookie, while I tried to make sense of Sang's rapid-fire chatter.

"We love Michael. Always put Michael first!"

But she emphasized that Helen and Mike were a dangerous combination, also that Mike had smacked Ron the previous week, and that families have to know the place is safe for their loved ones.

She started talking even faster.

"Helen not even incontinent. Family pays $4,800 a month. Not about money! Not about money! You like Green Hill Care Home. Wait. You see. Beautiful, sparkling clean tile floors! Better than here! Citrus Heights. Little bit closer. Not about money! We love Mike! Have 30 days before move. Plenty time! October 4."

Sang pointed to the date already circled on the wall calendar, then started all over again. They loved Mike. He and Helen were dangerous together. Not about money. Not about money. Daniel was nowhere to be seen.

Marg and I visited Green Hill Care Home. It was on level ground with a broad cement walkway leading to the front door. A border of straggly, water-starved plants lined the walkway. No hill. No greenery. Who names these places anyway?

We met with the caregiver/co-administrator, Livia, whom we immediately liked. Livia, her mother, Elena, and a live-in helper usually shared caregiving and maintenance tasks, though because Livia was five months pregnant, she would soon be less available. Elena, Green Hill's owner/co-caregiver, would take over the main responsibilities in a few weeks, when she returned from visiting family in Romania. Livia's husband helped out before and after work, as needed, and would continue to do that. Their two boys, 9 and 11, were both were thrilled by the prospects of a new baby brother or sister.

Green Hill itself was gleaming clean and much more orderly than Sang's, though none of this would, we thought, make any difference to Mike. There were only two other residents, both women, and neither was ambulatory. It was highly unlikely that anyone would get in Mike's way there. Livia assured us that Mike would be fine with them. It turned out that Sang had actually brought Mike to visit there a few weeks back, and Livia had been to Sister Sarah's two or three times to see Mike at "home."

It seemed Sang and Livia had already established that Green Hill Care Home would be a good placement for Mike. Apparently Sang had been working on this for a month or so. However, Mike's eviction from Sister Sarah's would have been a less bitter pill to swallow had I been in on it from the beginning.

Marg and I agreed that Mike might possibly do okay at Green Hill Care Home.

The day after we visited Green Hill, I got a call that a nearby three-tiered facility, Winding Creek (again, no curves, no creek), had an opening for an ALW resident. I'd visited this place several times—early on when I'd first started looking at memory care facilities, and again when I realized that Mike's situation at The Guiding Star was precarious. On each visit I was impressed with the director and with her empathy for dementia patients. She, Anna, assured me that they dealt with a number of FTD patients, and she was certain they could deal with Mike.

Winding Creek's fees for memory care were more than $6,000 a month, but they did have four ALW spaces. There was always a waiting list for those "beds," though, and their own high-paying residents got first dibs when an ALW space opened up. I'd put Mike on their waiting list months before he was kicked out of The Guiding Star and now, miracle of miracles, Mike was next in line for the bed that had just become available.

Mike had already been evaluated and approved by a nurse with the ALW program, but he also needed approval from Winding Creek's RN. I was hopeful. We were all hopeful. The visit was scheduled for the next day.

Mike was not on his best behavior when the Winding Creek nurse showed up. It was lunchtime, and everyone but Mike was eating around the kitchen table. When Mike walked by on his loop, he slowed down long enough to reach for Ron's plate. Ron held on. Mike jerked the plate away and yelled, "Fuck you!" He took a few bites of sandwich, set the plate on the bookshelf, and walked on.

When I talked with Anna later, she was apologetic. The nurse didn't approve Mike's application.

"Ours wouldn't be a good placement for him."

"But you manage with other FTD residents?"

"I know. But your Michael is extreme."

The next morning I drove to Green Hill Care Home and gave Livia a check for $2,800 for Mike's first month's rent.

On the morning of October 3, I picked Mike up from Sister Sarah's and took him for a long ride, during which time Dorin, Livia's husband, with help from Dale and Daniel, loaded up his van with Mike's belongings and delivered them to Mike's new room. Dale took some of the overflow.

As I walked Mike to the car on his last day at Sister Sarah's, Sang came close to me for a hug.

"You love me!" she said. "I know you love me!"

"Not exactly," I told her, stepping back. "But I'll always be grateful to you for all you've done for Mike and for the excellent care you've provided for him."

I opened the passenger side door. Mike got in and buckled up. He still buckled up. I got in on my side, checked to be sure the child lock was engaged, and drove away.

2013

Dear Mike,

I wish you would stop walking your loop long enough to sit beside me on the couch at Sister Sarah's. Sit and let me talk to you. I'd like to tell you that I'm sorry I was always a few steps behind in realizing the progression of your illness, expecting things from you that you could no longer give, being angered by your anger when you must have felt so lost and confused that anger was all you had left. I'm sorry I wasn't more gentle with you when you refused to shower, or insisted on putting on your tuxedo for a nonexistent concert, or disappeared in the supermarket.

I'd like to tell you that I'm sorry I couldn't take care of you 24/7. Sometimes I look at Sang and think, if she can do it, with six residents, why can't I do it just with you? But I couldn't physically keep track of you 24/7, and you were always angry, more angry with me than with anyone, I think, though you never smacked me the way you've smacked other caregivers. But here's the other thing, too: I was becoming so worn down and depleted, it seemed that if there weren't some relief, our kids would be losing not just one but both of their parents. No matter how hard I tried, I couldn't make things better for you. There is a poem by Mary Oliver, "The Journey," that tells of the narrator's struggle to finally leave other demands behind, to move on, and to save the only life he/she had the power to save. I found wisdom and solace in "The Journey."

But although I'm no longer with you 24/7, I'd like to tell you that I will always watch out for you. I will always make sure you're getting good care. I will always visit you, and bring you cookies, and check to see that all is well—as well as it can be, given the circumstances.

I'm certain that even if you stopped looping long enough for me to say all of these things to you, the words wouldn't reach you. But I'd like to say them to you anyway. I'd like the illusion of letting you know how I feel, how hard I've tried and am trying.

I don't think you would understand a word of such talk, but I'd like to say it all to you, anyway. As it is, the letters, another illusion, will have to do.

Marilyn

FOOT PROBLEMS

October through December 2013

W hen Sang got Mike dressed in the mornings, she'd always put shoes on him. By mid-morning, though, he was usually barefoot.

"It okay, honey, no fight with Mr. Mike over shoes."

He had several pair of shoes at Sang's, but the shoes he was wearing the morning we took him to Green Hill were worn-out red sneakers that were not his. I rummaged through the clothing in his "new" room to find another pair of shoes and, with the help of cookies and cajoling, we managed to get him to sit still long enough to take the old shoes off. He took his socks off on his own and resumed his loop.

The brief glimpse I got of his bare feet was shocking. They had apparently not been washed for some time. Mike always looked clean when I visited him at Sang's, but how could his feet be so dirty if he was being showered daily? Worse than that, his toenails were grossly overgrown and ringed by dried blood.

"Not good," Livia said. "We'll work on his feet this evening, when Dorin can help."

Livia was quite attentive to Mike and turned out to be good at figuring out what worked best for him and what didn't. Her husband showered Mike in the mornings. She said Mike loved Dorin. There was no telling whether or not he missed Sang and Daniel. The secure yard at Green Hill was much smaller than Sang's, and although Mike's loop was shorter than before, he seemed to have adapted to the new space. By the end of the first week, Mike was sleeping in his bed, usually from around 10 at night until 4 in the morning, when he got up and started walking. At Sang's Mike only wanted to sleep on the couch, and even then his sleep was more sporadic. So far, things were better than I had expected.

Shortly after the move, I stopped by Sang's to pick up some papers I'd forgotten on moving day. Sang gave a lengthy monologue justifying/explaining why Mike needed to move and why the new place was a good choice. I still felt that I was not getting the whole picture. I am not likely ever to fully understand the sudden need to move Mike, but it was senseless to stew about that. They took Mike on when he was in an extremely difficult phase and managed him with respect, grace, and humor. I needed to appreciate that, even though I would continue to be confused by the sudden eviction.

The feel of the two places was quite different. Sister Sarah's was always clean enough. Green Hill was consistently spotless. At Sister Sarah's, Mike could wander through the kitchen whenever he wanted. The refrigerator was secured shut with a latch, as were many of the cupboards. But the ones that were not Mike-proofed he could open and rummage around in, sometimes grabbing a handful of crackers, taking a few bites, depositing them here and there along the way.

At Green Hill, Elena didn't want Mike in the kitchen and, shortly after he moved in, she blocked both entrances to the kitchen with something akin to child gates, but harder to open.

At Sister Sarah's, Sang handed food to Mike as he walked through on his loop, or sometimes left food on one of the shelves where he himself often deposited food. He ate continuously at Sang's. At Green Hill, Elena wanted Mike to eat at the table with the rest of them, at regular mealtimes. She might put a bowl of Cheerios within reach, or a stack of crackers on a plate, but "real" food was offered at set mealtimes, at the table.

When Elena led Mike to the table, he would sit long enough to take a huge bite of whatever was there, then get back to his loop. He would, though, walk past the table for more food until it was gone. He would also, fairly often, grab food from someone else's plate. It seemed he was ravenous, even though at both places his food intake was prodigious.

He weighed 190 when he left The Guiding Star. He was around 160 when he entered Green Hill.

Two weeks after Mike moved in, he hit Sandy, the live-in caregiver. She told Livia she couldn't work with Mike and quit on the spot. She gave no notice, just walked away. As difficult as the immediate loss of help was, Livia took it in stride. Within days she'd hired another live-in caregiver, though it would be two weeks before that person could start. Livia had worked with this person before, and thought she'd do well with Mike.

Every move required a new doctor's report, so before the 30-day time period passed, Livia and Dorin took Mike to a 7:30 doctor's appointment with Dr. Weston, his new doc. Livia had worked with Dr. Weston with other residents and felt that he was responsive. We had no real connection with the Medi-Cal doctor Mike had been seeing for the past year or so, so the shift was easy. Dr. W. was closer, seemed thorough, and understood that we would not be treating anything except for comfort and pain relief, so he was an okay match.

When they saw the doctor, Livia asked to try Mike on Paxil. They'd had good responses with that drug with other residents and were hoping to find something that would have a calming effect on Mike. He had recently been slightly more agitated than usual, shoving Elena when she was trying to clean him up, sometimes purposefully banging his arm against a doorjamb as he went through. He continued smacking anyone who got in his way or who tried to get him to do anything. Apparently increased agitation is sometimes the case during the first few weeks adjusting to Paxil, before the more desired result kicks in. I didn't have much faith in anything helping to calm Mike, since we'd tried so many things in the past, including Paxil, to no avail. But, of course, I was willing to give it a try if Livia/Elena thought it could help.

Sharon came for a quick overnight to visit Mike in the new place. He was, very briefly, overjoyed to see her.

In the fall of 2011, in my other life, I had signed on as a volunteer with 916 Ink, a fledgling nonprofit dedicated to increasing Sacramento youth literacy through creative writing. My first and second semesters of volunteering consisted of 12 weeks of three-hour stints, on Fridays, at a local charter school. The official teacher with whom I was volunteering was one of those bright, caring, energetic, creative teachers that, if cloned, could fix all of the nation's shortcomings in education. Having taught high school English for 22 years, I had my own bag of tricks. But I learned a whole lot from Teacher B, especially in the realm of how to prime the creative juices of unconfident writers. Not only that, it was great fun.

During the course of the 12 weeks, students wrote poetry, fiction and creative nonfiction. They then chose a few of their favorite pieces and, with the help of an official editor, they worked on revision. Their works were then published in a professionally produced anthology. There followed a book release party, with readings, sales, and autographs. It was amazing to watch the transformation of mostly shy, doubtful writers into confident published authors.

Because my heart is with the underserved, and because I'd done some work with Sacramento Juvenile Hall residents some time back, I was able to start a 916 Ink program at that facility. For that work I would receive a stipend from the county office of education. It was not enough to bridge the negative gap between income and outgo, but it could add a few extra months to the hit-rock-bottom timeline.

In mid-October, shortly after Mike's move to Green Hill, I'd written in my journal:

I'm feeling good about the recent work I've done with the Juvenile Hall girls. Their writing is not sophisticated, but it's honest and raw, and I think the book will turn out well. After a break of a month or so I'll start with a group of boys.

It's good to expand my horizons and to have more on my mind than Mike, Mike, Mike. Not that I want to ignore him, but to think about him only 12,573 times a day, rather than 16,840, doesn't really lessen my concern. And to focus 4,267 daily thought-times on incarcerated girls offers a break in the thought-streaming. Also, they like knowing that I think about them even when not in their presence. It can't hurt.

That first book, *Caught Up*, offered a real boost to the writers. For some, it was the first time their voices had ever been valued. For others, seeing their work in print was a vote of confidence. I've since been a part of the publication of three more books from Juvenile Hall, and one from students, mostly on probation, in a group home.

As heartbreaking as it is to witness young lives in such disarray, I love seeing these writers grow in skill and confidence.

In late October, Elena returned from her extended family visit in Romania. Her English skills were more limited than Livia's, and her accent more pronounced, making communication with her more of a challenge. But, as was true of Livia, it was obvious that Elena was also strongly committed to making things work with Mike.

Neither Livia nor Elena had started out thinking they would be caregivers when they grew up. Livia had worked for the government in Romania, in an administrative capacity. Elena had taught first grade. When they came to the U.S., they both took entry-level jobs as caregivers in assisted living/dementia establishments because that was the only work that was available to them. Both said that in spite of their early trepidation, they came to love the work.

They were typical of a vast number of immigrants, from the Philippines, Ukraine, Latin America, Mexico, the Caribbean, and, as with Sang, Southeast Asia. They started out grossly underpaid, doing the dirtiest of the dirty work and some, like Sang, Livia and Elena, became successful entrepreneurs while offering a much-needed service.

The person Elena had planned to hire couldn't get her schedule worked out, so they continued the search for another live-in caregiver.

Sunny and Mike didn't pay much attention to each other anymore. A brief look from him, a quick sniff from her, and they each went their separate ways, but I liked to take her with me sometimes, and Sang never objected.

At first Elena was hesitant to have Sunny visit there, but after the first month gave her okay. The first time I took Sunny to Green Hill, one of the usually silent women, Kate, brightened when she saw her.

"What's your doggie's name?" she asked, leaning forward to better see the dog.

"Sunny," I said.

"Cute doggie," she said.

Although Kate was usually awake and sitting in the living room whenever I visited, that was the first time I'd seen her smile, or heard her speak.

I led Sunny over close to where she was sitting. Mike stopped by my side.

"Cute doggie, Sunny," she said, again with a broad smile.

I always carried treats in my pocket for Sunny, in case I had to lure her into the car, or get her to stand still while I attached her leash. I handed Kate a few treats, assuring her that Sunny wouldn't bite.

"Here, Sunny," she said holding a treat out in front of her.

Mike lunged, grabbed the treat, popped it into his mouth, chewed vigorously, and swallowed it almost as quickly as Sunny would have. Although dog treats may not have been part of the good nutrition plan, I was pretty sure it wouldn't hurt him.

After weeks on Paxil, I didn't see any changes with Mike one way or the other. He still lashed out when either Elena or the newly hired caregiver tried to get him cleaned up.

Elena reassured me that they were fine. "Don't worry," she said, whenever I expressed my concern.

"Don't worry" might have been more reassuring had I not recently experienced Sang's repeated orders—don't worry, don't worry, don't worry—followed by a 30-day eviction notice.

Seeing Kate's response to Sunny, I'd vowed to bring her with me whenever I visited. However, my next visit included one of those self-imposed errand circuits, and I hadn't backtracked to pick her up before I went to Green Hill. Once there, I greeted Mike. He walked on but after a few minutes he came back inside and sat in a recliner facing the TV. I sat next to him. He was on my right, and Sunny's admirer was on my left.

"How's that Sunny doggie?" Kate asked.

I was surprised that she'd remembered Sunny's name. I told her that Sunny was home napping, but I'd be sure to bring her on my next visit.

"I want to see her," she told me. "I had a dog back when I lived as a human."

As strange as that phrase, "back when I lived as a human" was, when I considered Kate's present life, the phrase seemed apt.

Mike was back to his loop, and as he went out the door Kate said, "I worry about him sleeping outside all night, but they say he likes it."

"I think he's in and out during the night," I said.

"Sometimes we used to take our sleeping bags outside and sleep under the stars, back when I lived as a human," Kate said.

Mike had become more and more adamantly opposed to having his fingernails cut. Just after Thanksgiving, Sharon and I had tried to trim his nails, but he yanked his hand away before the first clip could be made. It was as if he were afraid of being cut. No matter how hard we tried to reassure him, he would have none of it. His nails had grown extremely long, and he had places on his arms where he'd scratched and drawn blood.

The Paxil, which we'd hoped would calm him, had no effect. If anything,

Mike had been slightly more agitated since he'd started on it. We were gradually weaning him off that medication, with the possibility of trying something else. The only things I'd ever seen calm him were so strong they'd nearly knocked him unconscious.

Early in December, while shopping for groceries, I reached for a quart of milk and saw an array of eggnog cartons on the adjoining shelf. It was the season. Fat free, light, the original recipe, organic, and with soy milk. I was reminded of how much Mike had loved eggnog, and, though knowing Elena would not approve, I grabbed a carton, the original recipe, and added it to my collection of broccoli, low fat milk, and toilet paper.

When Sunny and I visited the following day, I watched as Elena read the eggnog label carefully. She sighed and shook her head. I suggested that she let Mike have a very small portion and see how it went. She said she would, but I could see she was resistant to the idea. She was being very careful about what he ate and felt that the extreme diarrhea was slightly less frequent.

I liked to offer Mike a bit of pleasure by bringing a favorite food to him when I visit, but I needed to follow Elena's lead on this, since she was the one on cleanup duty. The soy latte Sharon brought Mike on her previous visit had received Elena's stamp of approval, so soy latte it was. Decaf, of course. Honestly, I didn't know if it made any difference to Mike. He downed whatever we handed him, and plenty we didn't.

When I entered on that eggnog day, Kate, the dog lover, was in her chair, staring off into space. She brightened. "I knew Sunny was coming," she said.

With my right hand I pulled a handful of Cheerios from my pocket for Mike. With my left I handed Kate a few doggie treats. That worked.

That evening I went to the Chanteuses Christmas concert—very nice music, well done. But as I sat there I couldn't help remembering Mike's better days, back when he was their director. I didn't want to, wouldn't ever, forget the Mike who was. On the other hand, the Christmas season was so filled with *that* Mike that I felt I needed to carefully portion my remembrances.

On the wall in my office I had a Cherokee proverb, "Don't let yesterday use up too much of today," advice that I needed to be particularly careful to heed during this time of year. It is a poignant time for all of us, so many precious holiday seasons stacked one upon the other in our memory files, so many visitations from past people and long-gone times. Like the eggnog, best to be taken in small doses.

TOOTH AND NAIL
December 2013 through March 2014

Just before Mike left Sang's, he'd lost two teeth. One when he bit into a cookie. Another that he just spit out onto the ground as I watched him walking his loop. His brushing techniques left much to be desired and, of course, he wouldn't allow anyone to help him. So it was no surprise when, a couple of weeks before Christmas, Elena had noticed that Mike's jaw was swollen and his lower right gum was inflamed. She'd given him ibuprofen and the swelling subsided, but it was soon back again. We knew he needed to be seen by a dentist, but we also knew he was unlikely to be cooperative. I wanted to take advantage of Matt's availability before he left town, since Mike was still more likely to be cooperative with Matt than with anyone else.

In discussing the difficulties of keeping Mike in a waiting room with others, how he needed to be constantly on the move, which generally included trying to get into examination rooms, or out the door to wherever, or out emergency exits, Dr. E , our longtime regular dentist, offered to meet us in his office on the Sunday after Christmas, days before Matt and family were scheduled to leave.

One of Dr. E's dental assistants also joined us. It continued to amaze me that so many people, both friends and professionals, were willing to go the extra mile under difficult circumstances.

At our request, and in hopes of keeping Mike calm, the dentist called in a prescription for Valium. Because it would take an hour or so for the pill to take effect, Matt and I got to Green Hill about an hour before Mike's appointment, gave him the Valium, and waited for it to start working. Marg was waiting for us in the dentist's parking lot and helped us get a very groggy, unstable Mike on his feet and into the office. He stayed seated in the dental chair, mostly on the verge of sleep, while Dr. E examined his mouth, then, with the help of his assistant, took X-rays. Matt, Marg and I were on the job, anticipating a difficult time, but our fears were, luckily, not fulfilled. Thank the Goddess for Valium.

A word here about Valium and other anti-anxiety drugs. There were meds that could tamp down Mike's combativeness, but they also caused him to be unsteady on his feet. Livia and Elena were opposed to those because, with Mike's constant looping, the likelihood of a fall would be greatly increased. I knew they were concerned with Mike's well-being, but they were also concerned about their reputation within the licensing bureaucracy. Falls in a facility raise red flags, and they definitely didn't want red flags.

The immediate dental problem was an abscessed gum, for which Mike would be treated with an antibiotic. But his mouth was a mess, with seven or eight broken-off teeth, and his gums were highly susceptible to infection. We wanted only the most conservative treatment to minimize infection and to keep Mike pain free, but what would "conservative treatment" mean?

As much as I would have liked to continue having Mike be treated by our regular dentist, Dr. E did not take Medi-Cal patients, and private dental work was way beyond my means. Dr. E recommended a consultation with an oral surgeon, so I needed to find a Medi-Cal dentist who could then refer me to a Medi-Cal oral surgeon.

After Internet searches, checking reviews, making numerous phone calls complete with Press 1 for …, Press 2 for …, Press 3 for …," then being held captive by static, tinny "music," minutes had accumulated to hours that felt like days. Finally, though, I made an appointment with a dentist who, judging from Internet reviews, was the lesser of several evils.

On the day of our appointment, Dorin drove Mike down to the office in his van equipped with childproof doors. Marg and I met them in the parking lot of the new dentist's building about 7:50 for the 8 o'clock appointment. Usually Mike would be doing anything possible to get out of the van, and one of us would have to walk some loop with him in the parking lot until the doors opened. That morning, though, he sat quietly in the van until we could get inside. The glories of Valium.

It turned out my fears about a Medi-Cal dentist were unfounded. The office was clean and cheerful. The staff understood our situation and got Mike set up with the dentist as quickly as they could, although "quickly as they could" wasn't quick enough for Mike. Dorin and Marg took turns walking Mike up and down the outer hallway while I finished the necessary reams of paperwork.

Once seated in the dental chair, Mike needed some prompting to stay there but, unlike Valium-free times, that was easily managed. The dentist was gentle, thorough, and sympathetic to our situation. He agreed that we should do as little as possible and started the paperwork for referral to an oral surgeon, recommending extraction of only the tooth that was most prone to infection.

The front desk woman was knowledgeable about Medi-Cal dental benefits and walked us through what we might expect of coverage for oral surgery.

By the time we left, the Valium was wearing off, and Mike was on his way back to restlessness and anxiety. But it had worked long enough. I dreaded his having to go through the next process. He would undoubtedly have to be anesthetized. As helpful as the Valium was for brief visits, oral surgery would be a whole other affair.

What followed was another round of phones calls, scanning and emailing power of attorney documents to the next office, repeating ID numbers, birthdates, what I'd had for breakfast and Sunny's maiden name. As tedious as this all sounds, it doesn't begin to depict the reality of tediousness.

Our appointment with the Medi-Cal oral surgeon was more difficult than had been our experience with the referring Medi-Cal dentist. Despite being assured by phone that staff would get Mike in quickly, we had an hour-and-a-half wait. During that time Mike was up and down, out the door, walking past other offices, trying to get into other offices, coming back into the dentist's office, leaning over the counter to look around, trying to get back to the treatment area, etc. Marg, Livia and I took turns walking with Mike, but it was an excruciatingly long and busy wait. When Mike finally got taken back to see the dentist, it took him all of five minutes to assess the situation. He felt it would be best to do the job with only a local anesthetic, with help from Valium. They would give Mike a 10:45 appointment, the first of the day, and get him right in so we could avoid the nerve-wracking wait.

The following week, a little before 10:45, Marg and I met Elena and Mike in the parking lot. Mike was somewhat subdued, having been given a Valium about 45 minutes before the scheduled extraction. Mike waited with Elena in her car while I checked to see if the dentist was ready for us. The front desk person gave me two forms to fill out, and took my cell phone number so she could call when the dentist was ready. I completed and waited for the phone call from the office. Mike was getting restless and, around 11 o'clock, I went back inside to check with the receptionist. She said the dentist was flying in from LA and should be there any time. She'd let me know.

At 11:30, after one or the other of us had completed many circles of the lot with Mike, 45 minutes after our "we'll get him right in" appointment, the dentist still wasn't there, nor had he been heard from. This was obviously not the oral surgeon for us. Mike's tooth/gum had not been bothering him for the past few weeks. Marg and I had been questioning the necessity of putting Mike through such a procedure anyway. We gave it up.

Though we'd managed to sidestep oral surgery, it was impossible to sidestep nail-clipping issues. Livia and Dorin had managed to clip Mike's fingernails and toenails days after he entered Green Hill back in October, but they'd had no success in future tries. By early February, the length and sharpness of Mike's fingernails was a danger to himself and to anyone else around him. He had scratches, some open, on both arms. Elena also had scratches from Mike's attempts to push her away during the course of daily hygiene necessities. After we endured several unsuccessful nail-clipping endeavors, Mike's doctor prescribed trazodone to be taken half an hour or so before the next try.

In a bow to the prohibition against caregivers cutting nails, I joined Elena, Livia and Dorin around 8 o'clock one evening, scissors and nail clippers in hand. By that time, the trazodone should have taken effect. Livia and Dorin's three sons were also there and the older boys entertained their baby brother while the adults got to work.

Mike had been in bed when I arrived, but he got up as soon as he saw me. He gave me a quick smile and started walking. I led him back to bed and suggested he stretch out. He did, for an instant, then tried to get up again. I sat on the bed in a position that made it difficult for Mike to get up.

My presence, with my nail-cutting tools, was mainly for show. I was more than happy that Livia, undoubtedly a more competent nail cutter than I, was on hand, complete with sterile gloves, cotton swabs, and alcohol.

Mike was definitely more relaxed under the influence of trazodone than he would otherwise have been, but "more relaxed" wasn't exactly relaxed enough. I sat facing him, blocking his view, talking to him, rubbing his neck and shoulders while holding his upper right arm secure. Dorin, the strongest of the gathering, secured Mike's lower arm, just above the wrist, in an attempt to keep him still enough for Elena to clip his nails. Elena stood beside the bed, reassuring Mike, or at least trying to, that we all loved him and that no one would hurt him.

At the first attempt to clip a nail, Mike jerked his hand away. We all went on with reassurances. Another attempt. Another jerking away. That was the pattern for what seemed like hours but was probably more like 15 long minutes. Finally, the right hand completed, we shifted positions to secure the left hand, to block Mike's view, and to continue our attempts at reassurance.

"Take a deep breath," I said, as Elena retrieved Mike's jerked away hand. In a doctor's office, Mike would still take a deep breath at a doctor's suggestion. However, my attempts to guide him into deep breathing fell short.

The toenails required another, more pronounced shift of positions. At one point Elena somehow ended up on my lap. Eventually the deed was done.

"All done, Mike," I told him. "Okay?"

He smiled, nodded, got out of bed, and started a loop. He walked around for five or so minutes, then went back to bed.

As I was leaving, Elena, a nondrinker, suggested that vodka might be more effective and less extreme than trazodone. What did I think? I said I thought anything was worth a try—use their own best judgment. What I didn't say was that I could hardly wait to get home to give myself a vodka treatment.

In my other world, I spoke at an English teacher's conference about engaging reluctant readers with material of their liking. I never tire of mounting that soapbox, and the talk was well-received.

New Wind Publishing had a table in the exhibit hall where we hawked books and talked with teachers, some of whom I'd known from years past. It was good to reconnect, and to be out in the broader world, especially since the weekend away had been free of emergency phone calls.

On a visit shortly after the nail-clipping caper, I managed to get Mike to stand still on Green Hill's scale long enough to get a reading: 130 pounds. Mike's weight loss was a mystery. He ate a lot, hour after hour, day after day. Perhaps it was the persistent diarrhea, or continually being in motion, or something else. All the basic tests—blood, urine and stool—had been given more than once, and nothing showed up to answer either the question of why weight loss or why diarrhea.

Mike remained amazingly strong given his low weight. He also showed no signs of being in pain. My main concern was that he not be in pain. An earlier major concern was that he not be fearful, or agitated, or anxious, but there'd been no solutions to those problems and at this stage, I doubted there would be.

By mid-April, Mike's weight was down to 124 pounds. Elena insisted that the scale was inaccurate. That was possible, maybe even likely, but it showed a trend. Elena told me, "He's gaining weight. He's getting fat around the middle."

"Really?"

"Yes. I shower him every day. Sometimes two or three times a day. He is gaining weight around the middle."

On the next round I caught Mike and rubbed his belly. There was a slight pooch at his waist, sort of like the very early stages of pregnancy.

"Getting a beer belly?" I asked.

Mike smiled and walked on.

His pooch was not high enough for a distended liver. At least I didn't think so. But I wondered, wouldn't he someday experience the sort of organ shutdown that got Karen Carpenter? How much more weight could he lose and still carry on?

On the lighter side, Elena called to Mike, "Come here. Show Marilyn" (pronounced Mary Lin) "your nails."

I followed as he walked past.

"Let's see your hand," I said, catching up and walking beside him. I held my hand out to him. He didn't take it. Gently, carefully, I reached for his hand. Before he yanked it back, I got of glimpse of nicely trimmed nails.

"How did you manage that?" I asked Elena.

"Livia and Dorin helped. Easy. It was bedtime. He was very relaxed."

I waited for her to say more. When she didn't, I asked, "Did you give him trazodone?"

"No."

"Valium?"

"No. No drugs. It was easy."

Recalling the wrestling match four of us had the last time Mike's nails had reached the length of Cruella De Vil's, it was hard for me to consider "easy." I pressed on.

"So how did you manage?"

"Just a little bit," she said, holding thumb and index finger less than an inch apart.

She watched intently for my reaction. "In 7-UP. Just a little."

It was then that I remembered the conversation she, Livia, and I had after the very difficult nail-cutting escapade back in February.

"Vodka?"

She nodded.

"Whatever it takes," I said.

She held a finger to her lips. "Shhhhh."

It was not only against regulations for caregivers to clip nails. It was definitely against regulations to dispense vodka. Elena was careful to follow the letter of the law, her livelihood held in the hands of licensing agency personnel. I did appreciate that, in times of desperation, she was willing to act beyond the proverbial box.

I was ever grateful for people like Elena and Sang. Even though our parting from Sang and Daniel was uneasy and strange, the care they gave Mike for more than a year was invaluable. Elena's style of caregiving was very different from Sang's, but she, too, was always on the job, practical, efficient, and affectionate.

Whenever I thought of Elena at work, I wondered how she could manage to do everything for three needy people when I had been unable to manage even for one. But after a walk, or music, or a glass of wine, I am comforted by the reminder that, given our own particular strengths and weaknesses, we all do what we can do.

ANOTHER LOSS

April 30, 2014

Sunny had been diagnosed with congestive heart failure back in January. Unlike her earlier self, she was ready to return from walks after just a few blocks, but she'd been doing well with the help of meds.

Then around 3 o'clock in the morning, Monday, April 30, I was awakened by her coughing, gagging and gasping for air. She scratched at the door to go outside, but balked at the two steps that led down from my kitchen into the patio. I carried her outside and set her down on the grass, thinking she needed to pee. But she just stood there, struggling to breathe. I took her back inside, put her on my bed, and lay down beside her. This was usually a place of comfort for her, but she struggled to get down and go back outside. Perhaps it was the cool air she wanted, or the slight breeze. Whatever it was, she stood gasping and heaving for breath. Nothing I could do relieved her distress.

I called the emergency vet. They recommended that I bring her in so they could give her an intravenous dose of Lasix, and oxygen for short-term relief. They confirmed, though, that the results of such treatment would be short-lived. The question was not only why would I put her through that, the long drive, the lonely medical procedures, but how could I afford such treatment?

I comforted her as best I could. I got her to our nearby regular vet as soon as they opened. By that time she was unable to walk and her struggle for every breath was even more severe. At that point the kind thing seemed to be to help her on her way. I held her close as the vet injected her with the drug that would ease her ending. Her body slowly relaxed, the struggle for breath ended, and she was gone. By the time I left the parking lot, I was missing her terribly. But I had no doubt that I'd made the right decision. Although her last few hours had been extremely difficult, she'd had a long, happy life, and was amazingly healthy until her last few months. Not bad for an old girl of 93 dog years.

She had been my alarm clock, regularly rousing me within 15 minutes on either side of 6:30. The Tuesday morning after that fateful Monday, about 6:15, still mostly asleep, I heard Sunny stirring, shaking her head and rattling her tags, just as I'd been hearing over the past 13 years, ever since we bought her first puppy collar, and secured her first license and identity tags. It took a moment to realize that the sounds I'd heard were only ghosts of the familiar—that Sunny now only lived in the realm of dreams and memory.

Would that I had been able to do for Mike what I'd done for Sunny. But Mike was destined to walk his anxiety-ridden loop, day in and day out, until something less certain and comfortable than the vet's potion relieved him of his tortured life.

HOSPICE CARE

April through July 2014

With guidance from Marg, I managed to get Mike connected with hospice care. He didn't meet the hospice "six months to live" criteria, but, because of his steady weight loss, he did fit the "failure to thrive" category. On that basis, Mike's doctor was willing to make a referral. Hospice took his case for 90 days, after which they would re-evaluate. The advantage of hospice care was that they provided added support—a weekly visit from a hospice nurse, visits with a social worker, and plenty of expert guidance. They would send a home health care worker to Green Hill three times a week. With Livia being less available because of the baby, and given their frustrating, fruitless search for a live-in caregiver, Elena needed all the help she could get. (Hospice also provided incontinence supplies, a savings to me of around $100 per month.)

While Mike was officially under the care of hospice, if there was an emergency, the folks at Green Hill would first call hospice rather than 911. Hospice would then make the decision about the next call. I knew they would avoid heroic measures. Without hospice, Green Hill would be required to call 911 given any emergency such as a fall or signs of a stroke. My biggest concern over that regulation was that, with the 911 rush to a hospital, in the heat of the moment, Mike's Physician Orders for Life-Sustaining Treatment that called for no heroic life-saving treatments might not be honored. The completed order was in his file at Elena's, ready to be handed off to any 911 responders. But I had heard too many horror stories of someone mistakenly being hooked up to a breathing device, or feeding tube, and the family then being unable to remove the devices. I didn't think any of that would be willful, but once the deed was done, it was not always possible to undo it. We could avoid such a dilemma with hospice on the job. They would assure that Mike be kept pain free, without any "heroic" measures. I didn't expect Mike to qualify for that program beyond the 90-day period, but it was good to have hospice on board for however long that could last.

At San Gabriel High School, the school where Mike taught music for 15 or so years before he retired in 1995, a ninth-grade "English Learner" teacher uses my books in his classroom. He's working to help his students develop a reading habit, and it turns out they're captivated by the stories in my Hamilton High Series. I heard about this from a district curriculum director who'd been at the conference I'd attended in February. Through her efforts, an author visit was arranged, and in May I made a quick trip to Southern California to talk with Mr. D's students. Though only a very few teachers remained from the days when Mike was there and when I was a frequent visitor, the campus still had a familiar feel to it.

I love talking with young readers about my books, the life of a writer, what they'd like to read about next, or anything else that comes up. All of the students in this group of ninth-graders, mostly Vietnamese, though a few Latino/a and Hmong, had read at least one of my books and several had read three or more. Two girls were adamant that I should have ended the novel *If You Loved Me* differently. We batted around other possible endings, I made a case for the ending as written, and all in all it was a lively, thought-provoking conversation.

During a break between presentations, the principal came in carrying three bulging albums he'd pulled from the archives, saying he thought I might like to have them. They chronicled choral events from 1987 to 1990. This principal had only been at SGHS for four years, so obviously he hadn't known Mike. Still, he somehow made the connection. I appreciated the gesture, though in reality I'd not been longing for more pictures. Nevertheless, a quick perusal of the albums reminded me of Mike's amazing accomplishments with young singers. After so many years of the diminished Mike, it's good to occasionally come across such reminders.

After I returned from Southern California, at the urging of the hospice nurse, Elena and I agreed to try Mike on an anti-anxiety medication. This was an effort to calm Mike so that he wouldn't be up and down all night long, and so he might be more manageable with showers and other basic hygiene needs. The results were what those of us who knew Mike expected. He became even more agitated than usual. After three days we went back to no meds.

As had been the case to one degree or another over the past four years,

Mike continued to smack caregivers as they tried to shower him, dress him, or sometimes just be within reach. He continued to yell, "Fuck you!" whenever he was irritated, and he was often irritated. Until this time, Mike's physical and verbal aggression had been limited to caregivers. Then, sometime in March, that changed.

On one of Marg's weekly visits, she caught up to the looping Mike on the patio. As always, he gave her a broad smile. He was carrying a CD, which he handed to her. When she took the offered CD, he smacked her hard on the hand. It was a quick smack, a sting that left no bruise or physical discomfort. But it took its toll. Marg, Mike's ongoing, stalwart supporter—although she continued visiting regularly—was left feeling less connected to Mike.

Mike had never before lashed out physically at any family member. The old Mike would have been appalled by the very idea of hitting Marg. What a cruel ending for such a bright, funny, talented, warm-hearted man.

On May 25, Mike's 74th birthday, I stopped at the market for more cookies and picked up a generic card for him. At Elena's, after Mike's first two cookie-grabbing rounds, I held the card out for him. He smiled, tore open the envelope, then set the card on one of the shelves where he often left things.

Subei had posted on Facebook a picture of the two of them, probably taken 12 or so years back when she was around 5. Mike was leaning against the kitchen island, on which sat flour, sugar, a big mixing bowl and other ingredients. He was beaming down at Subei, who was standing on a stool that put her in reach of the island top. She was holding a large spoon, her face smeared with what appeared to be chocolate, beaming back. Below the picture she'd written:

A happy, happy birthday to my dearest grandfather! Thank you for making me always feel like royalty, even when I wasn't really acting like it. Now let them eat cake!

I'd taken my iPad to show him Subei's picture and message. He gave it a quick glance and was on his way.

By early June Mike was down from 124 pounds to 120 pounds.

Toward the end of July, Mike's Florida niece, Beth, was with us for a week. She'd visited every summer since Mike's 2009 diagnosis. She and Mike had had a long, close connection. The changes she saw in him annually were much more dramatic than the changes the rest of us noticed on a more regular basis. For the first time Mike hadn't recognized Beth when she greeted him. It was no longer obvious to me that he recognized me either—the signs of recognition had become less and less obvious.

Cindi came in from Reno for a few days while Beth was in town. Once again, the Dodsons' place was party central, with dinners on their deck and plenty of levity in the midst of a shared awareness of loss and sorrow.

The day after Cindi's arrival, she, Beth, and I, went to see Mike at Green Hill. We found him standing on the patio, peering in through the glass door that led from the patio/yard into the house. I rushed to the door, unlocked it, and let him in. Usually slow to anger, I was enraged. Why was the door locked? It was 90-plus degrees outside! How long would he have been locked out in the heat of the day had we not arrived when we did?

The person to whom I was ranting, a new caregiver, spoke very little English, though she did understand tone and body language.

We led Mike to his room where we tried in vain to engage him with talk of pictures on the wall, albums on the chest, a stack of cards in a basket. In the midst of this, the caregiver came in and handed me a cell phone with Elena on the other end. Elena was talking about an emergency, but, just as I'd experienced with Sang, when Elena was anxious or stressed she talked so rapidly I could only catch a word here and there. I couldn't make sense of anything she was saying, but she definitely knew what I was saying. It was totally unacceptable to lock Mike outside at any time, even more so in the heat of a more than 90-degree day.

In truth, Mike didn't seem distraught and was none the worse for wear. Nevertheless, to find him locked out on a Sacramento summer day was alarming. Although no place was perfect, and there were times I might have wished that Elena was a little less rigid, I had never before doubted that Mike was being well cared for at Green Hill. Besides keeping Mike locked outside, what else had been going on that I'd been unaware of?

An hour or so after we returned from that disturbing visit, Livia called to explain the circumstances. She apologized over and over. She knew that was unacceptable, it was the only time it had ever happened, and it would never happen again. What I sensed in both Livia and Elena was the fear that I would file a complaint. Such a situation could lead to the loss of their license, something that would turn their lives and the lives of their families upside down.

What had happened was that while Livia and her family were on vacation in Southern California, their house had been broken into and robbed. Since Elena was the contact person, the police had called her and asked that she come immediately to Livia's house. Elena first said she couldn't do that right then, but the police insisted. Although neither Elena nor Livia said anything about this aspect of the experience, I knew that insistence of police with an immigrant from Romania carried an implicit threat beyond anything many American citizens would have experienced.

Elena told the caregiver that she had to leave, but she'd be back as soon as possible. The caregiver told Elena, "If you leave, I leave. I'm not staying here with him [Mike] on my own." I understood the dilemma and, to be honest, there had been times under my watch when, out of desperation, I'd traded safe practices for a few minutes of solitude, like sending Mike on errands when, in my heart of hearts, I'd known he shouldn't be driving.

In following conversations, both Elena and Livia assured me that they could handle Mike and that they wanted to continue to work with him. However, they also often reminded me of how difficult he was and that his behavior had made it difficult to keep any help. The most recent caregiver, the recipient of my rant, walked out as soon as Elena returned from her meeting with the police. Three others before her had quit. I could see that the demands of caring for Mike were wearing them down. I didn't know what would be next for him, but I needed to be considering other possibilities, just in case.

As a result of Leesa's urging, combined with her organizational skills, early July found us frolicking in Sunriver, Oregon, on an extended family vacation. Sharon, Doug, Lena, Subei, Dale, Marg, Corry, Matt and Leesa, cousin Linda and her partner Barb, Cindi and I, hiked, lolled about, went to the river, kayaked, white river rafted, swam, ate, drank, told stories, played Scrabble, watched soccer and generally carried on. It was a weeklong, wonderful combination of people and activities, thankfully free of Mike-related emergency calls. I returned home, refreshed and renewed, ready to tackle whatever compelling tasks needed to be tackled. I wasn't sure what those next tasks would be, but I was sure they *would* be.

As was expected, Mike was dropped from hospice care after 90 days. All of the people connected with hospice had been attentive and helpful, and I had particularly appreciated long conversations with Betty, the social worker, as she delved more deeply into possibilities of Assisted Living Waiver programs and other facilities that could offer some financial relief. Unfortunately, every place she suggested was closed to Mike because of his volatile behavior. If he had been wheelchair-bound, such places could deal with him, but because he was so mobile and strong, none of them would take him on. On her last visit to Mike, as his case was being closed out, she brought information on Priority Care, a behavioral health program that was connected with a local hospital.

"They sometimes have success with difficult patients," she said.

"I don't have much hope for that," I said.

"Honestly, I don't either," she said. But there's an outside chance, and it can't hurt. Medi-Cal will cover it."

I called the number on the card Betty left with me and set up a time for visits from the Priority Care psychiatric nurse and social worker. They completed an evaluation and the nurse recommended a new combination of drugs. That was tricky, though, because of Elena's resistance to having Mike on meds of any kind. I could have insisted, but I didn't want to go to war with Elena. She continued to assure me that they—mostly she—could manage Mike, but each time she reported that he'd smacked her or someone else, I saw that she was increasingly worn thin by his behaviors.

After a few weeks of visits and recommendations from Priority Care staff, we all realized that their attentions were exercises in futility, since, barring an out-and-out battle with Elena, there could be no follow through on Priority Care's recommendations.

Mike continued walking, walking, walking. He'd walk outside, then immediately come back inside. He went from one room to the next, picking things up, putting them down, sometimes moving them into another room. Kate, the one who'd had a dog back when she was a human, had been quite upset that her precious family picture album had gone missing. Then one day, weeks after its disappearance, I found it tucked away in the bottom drawer of Mike's chest.

Later in the summer of our Sunriver family vacation, Matt and Mika flew down for a short visit. Mike recognized Matt with a big smile and a quick hug, and walked on.

Between the two of us, Matt and I managed to get Mike to stand on the scale long enough to get a reading—115 pounds. Down five pounds from mid-June. He was apparently getting no benefit from the copious amounts of food he ate. He looked as if he were starving to death, and he ate as if he were starving, even going so far as to eat a hunk of foam rubber from a new patient's helmet.

In addition to calling the doctor, who was not immediately available—"if this is a life threatening situation, hang up and dial 911"—I Googled "eating foam rubber." It turned out there are people who crave foam rubber. Some went as far as to eat huge amounts of foam rubber from couch cushions. One woman confessed she was no longer welcome in a friend's house because she "ate her couch." I decided not to worry about the now seemingly small hunk of foam rubber Mike had ingested.

In my other life, before Subei returned to Kenyon College in Ohio as a sophomore, she came to my place for an overnight. We talked about anything and everything, ate Mexican food, went to Planet Earth Rising for a "spiritual adjustment"—an interesting experience neither of us expected to ever repeat. As part of an ongoing family tradition, we met Dale for breakfast at the Pancake Circus, a place with delicious waffles, vintage clown decor, and bad coffee. A perfect combination of send-off activities for my college sophomore granddaughter.

It was just after Labor Day when Mike, reaching for a cup of water, lost his balance and fell. He hit his head on the floor, gashed his head open, got up and kept walking. Livia called me immediately but my phone wasn't turned on. Because of Mike's situation I was diligent about keeping my phone on, charged and handy, but this one time …

Mike's head was bleeding. He wouldn't stop to let Livia see the extent of the damage. Livia called 911, EMTs came, and Mike was taken to the nearby emergency hospital. In the meantime, since she couldn't reach me, Livia called Dale and Marg. By the time I thought to check my phone and checked my messages (about 20 minutes after Livia called), Dale and Marg were at the hospital with Mike. He was already in a small room, in a hospital gown, propped up in a hospital bed.

The wound on Mike's head was not of a size or depth to warrant emergency treatment, but Livia and Elena didn't know that when they called 911. By the time I arrived on the scene, Mike had been seen by a doctor and was scheduled for a CT scan. About half an hour after I got there, an orderly came to wheel Mike down to the wing where he would get the scan. I walked along with them and waited with Mike. He was loosely confined but could still swing his legs over the side of the gurney. "Not yet," I kept telling him as I repositioned his legs onto the gurney. The CT showed no broken bones. The doctor said the gash would heal faster with two butterfly stitches, unless Mike was likely to pull them out. We skipped the butterflies.

The emergency wing of the hospital was extremely busy, a place definitely in need of more staff and more rooms. But the RNs, LVNs, doctors and orderlies, were all quick, competent, pleasant and friendly.

The examining doctor strongly recommended that Mike spend the night in the hospital for observation. But why? It was miserable for Mike to be confined in a hospital bed, unable to walk around freely, and it was also miserable and difficult for us to keep him in the bed. When the admitting doctor came to complete the paperwork for Mike's overnight stay, I told him we weren't going to do that. After trying to talk with Mike a bit, and watching us trying to get him to stay in the bed, the doctor agreed with our decision. I signed the release papers, which he approved. Dale and I took Mike back to Green Hill, while Marg returned home to get back to whatever she'd been doing when they got the call.

Livia and Elena did what they needed to do in calling 911, but life would have been easier for everyone had that call not been made.

Immediately after the hospital escapade, I requested that hospice reassess Mike in the hopes that, as before, he would qualify on the basis of his ongoing weight loss. Again Mike was approved because of his "failure to thrive." Next time, if there was a next time, hospice would make the 911 call decision.

By the end of that September, Mike's nails again needed major attention. Although the previous clipping had gone fairly smoothly, he'd been more agitated than usual during the following day. Elena and Livia were reluctant to use the vodka helper again. But when I mentioned the nail dilemma during a routine doctor's visit, the nurse practitioner said, "We can cut his nails. It won't be pretty, but we can do it." I made an appointment for the following week.

Marg and I met Livia and Mike at the office. As requested, I brought my own nail clippers. Mike sat in a chair. I sat on his lap, gripping the back of the chair in an attempt to keep him from bolting. Livia sat at Mike's left, hanging onto his left arm and hand to keep him from batting the clippers away. Marg worked at holding Mike's right arm and wrist secure, and the nurse practitioner struggled to clip his nails. She was right. It wasn't pretty. There was a lot of struggling—a lot of bucking and jerking around. Finally, though, the deed was done.

As frantic as Mike was during the process, as soon as he was released from our bondage, he seemed as fine as he ever seemed those days.

"That's a job well done," I told him, smiling. He nodded and smiled back as he opened the door to wherever his feet would take him next. The experience of fighting him and holding him down stayed with the rest of us for far too long, but I didn't think that was the case for Mike. We were all relieved to have the nails taken care of for a while, but the ones who dealt with Mike daily, physically, were particularly relieved to be free of scratches for a while.

By mid-October, Elena and Livia's desire to see Mike on his way had become a frequent topic of conversation. Green Hill had three new residents, two of them mobile with walkers. With those additions Mike had to be watched even more carefully. He'd already hit one of the new people as she made her way from her chair to the dining room.

"Too much," Elena said.

I couldn't blame her, and I appreciated not getting a 30-day ultimatum, but finding another place became even more urgent than when the main issue was "only" the ongoing money drain. With Janell, the new hospice social worker on the job, our search for a Medi-Cal facility was re-energized.

In my other life, I was thrilled that New Wind Publishing had reissued all 10 of my "True-to-Life Series from Hamilton High" books with fresh new covers and a new dedication to getting the books into the hands of high school students. Between the recession, the diminished promotional efforts of my previous publisher, and the responsibilities for Mike's care, my recent involvement in conferences for educators was negligible. That fall I was invited to speak to a group of school librarians. These librarians are mostly unsung heroes in the fight for literacy. They maintain and add to collections that appeal to readers of all levels and interests. They deal with efforts at censorship with courage and integrity, and with high rates of success. I jumped at the chance to be part of their upcoming conference.

Just moments after I'd agreed to their offer, I wished I hadn't. I was rusty. I was old. I was dull. But, except for divorcing my first husband, I never break an agreement, so I plunged forward.

It was gratifying to reconnect with librarians I'd known in the past, and to meet new ones. To hear what new books teens were gravitating toward (still a lot of vampires), and to learn that the Hamilton High books continued to draw readers. Since the very first book, it has never ceased to thrill me to hear a story of how one of my books was the first one a student had ever read, and how he/she came begging for more, and I heard that more than once on that occasion. For a few hours my mind and heart were lifted beyond the heartbreak of FTD, and the emptiness of my once full-of-life husband. For a few hours I didn't worry about money or the uncertain and necessary move from Green Hill. I wanted more such times.

In person, Janell visited numerous local facilities and a few that were not so local. The ones she didn't visit in person she contacted by phone. When I told her how much I appreciated her perseverance, she brushed it off, saying that because she was new to the area she needed to familiarize herself with as many memory care facilities as possible. It turned out that the only place in Sacramento that would consider taking an ambulatory patient with Mike's behaviors was North Point, the place we had considered before placing Mike at Sister Sarah's. North Point was large and institutional, housing about 170 patients. It served not only those with dementia and/or physical disabilities—it had a number of younger patients suffering from PTSD, and others with mental illnesses that made it impossible for them to live in more open settings. Through a combination of therapy, behavioral modification and drugs, they managed a wide range of behavioral difficulties. I was hopeful that something might finally be done to alleviate my poor husband's ongoing, severe anxiety.

Mike would be in a room with two to four others. His caregivers would be on a rotation system—very different than dealing with the same two people every day, as he did at Green Hill. On the other hand, North Point had two doctors and a psychiatrist who visited regularly. And although they tried to keep drugs to a minimum, they were experienced at prescribing and adjusting meds to deal with behavioral issues.

I'd been reluctant all along to have Mike in a less personal setting, dealing with a wide variety of caregivers rather than the same one or two he saw daily. But he now seemed less and less aware of his surroundings. I wondered if, at this stage, such a change would make much difference to him. I knew it would make a difference to me, going to visit Mike, walking down a wide hall lined with people strapped into wheelchairs, some slumped, heads as low as they could go, asleep or nodding off. Others, also strapped into wheelchairs, were calling out for help, or for Mommy, or for some other person known only to them. A few walked the halls. Some were quite pleasant. Many were distraught.

North Point's saving grace was the gently affectionate way that staff interacted with residents. The director seemed to know everyone by name, and he exchanged greetings with each person as he led the way down the hall to his office.

I was slowly coming to terms with the likelihood that Mike's next placement would be in a highly institutionalized setting. Within a few days of my North Point visit, Dale, Marg, and Sharon, all at different times, took the tour. Matt flew down from Walla Walla so he, too, could weigh in on the place again.

It was during another two martini cocktail hour that we accepted what seemed to be inevitable. None of us wanted to move Mike into North Point, but the only other places that might possibly take him were of the $10,000-a-month luxury memory care ilk. As it was, at $3,200 a month, I figured I had less than a year to go before every last penny of the remaining retirement account was used up. Then what? Even though I was an active, healthy 79, a return to full-time teaching didn't seem feasible. Three hours a week for 12 weeks at a time with a juvenile hall unit, plus preparing that unit's writing for publication, was one thing. Preparing for and teaching five high school English classes five days a week, plus reading and commenting on somewhere around 175 essays each week, was another. That task was tough enough at the age of 30. Besides, what principal in his/her right mind would hire a 79-year-old with so many teachers in their 20s and 30s looking for work?

We comforted one another that the North Point staff was warm and friendly, and it didn't smell too bad. From the comfortable, well-appointed Guiding Star, with private rooms and baths, with tasty food served in a spacious dining room, through the funkily but cheerfully decorated Sister Sarah's, to the more sparse but squeaky clean Green Hill, to North Point's drab, institutionalized hallways with rooms shared by up to six patients, our requirements and expectations had, out of necessity, changed. North Point was a no-aquarium, not-even-a-fish-bowl place, and we would be lucky to have Mike there.

As I drifted off to sleep after martinis, and dinner, after shared sadness and loss and resignation, the thought crossed my mind that the money drain might be checked, that the red figures at the end of each month might possibly turn to black. It was just a fleeting thought. Given my recent failed experiences with the waiver program and subsidized housing, I knew better than to court dreams of eased finances. Good thing.

In theory, North Point would accept Mike, but in practice there was road-block after roadblock. For one thing, Mike would be entering under a hospice plan. North Point had only eight hospice beds, and they were all taken.

Janell, the hospice social-worker gem, called North Point regularly to check on availability and to remind them of Mike's needs. She, the hospice nurse, and one of the hospice directors, met with the admissions director. Hospice even offered to provide on-site in-service training, with a focus on caring for Mike. The admissions director was impressed.

When a hospice bed opened, we expected it to be Mike's. But the North Point executive director was concerned that hospice would decertify Mike, leaving him unfunded. The hospice nurse, doctor, and social worker visited Mike and recertified him. Now at 112 pounds, he continued to meet the "failure to thrive" category.

With the threat of decertification removed, we assumed that the newly available hospice bed to be Mike's, but oops—North Point needed a lab test to show that Mike's diarrhea was not the result of a C. diff (Clostridium difficile) infection. The hospice doctor was sure that Mike did not have C. diff, but was nonetheless obtaining the test.

Then I got word that, based on Mike's behavior, the North Point staff had decided that they couldn't manage him. His unpredictable lashing out, his practice of taking food from others, his consistent, angry, physical resistance to showers, nail clipping, shaving, or any other physical hygiene efforts, all combined to bar him from the place that had seemed to take everyone. The director claimed that his hands were tied. It was a staff decision that included the director of nursing and caregiver representatives.

Hospice again met with the director of admissions, but North Point wouldn't budge. It seemed there was no facility in the greater Sacramento area willing to take Mike given his present behavior, and, because of Green Hill's concern about Mike's possible falling, we couldn't try him on any anti-anxiety drugs while he was there unless I hired someone 24/7 to be sure he didn't fall. It was financially impossible for me to provide 24-hour care for Mike. So we couldn't try to get Mike on an effective anti-anxiety drug while he was there. And facilities that can manage drug treatment wouldn't take him as long as his anxiety had him acting out. And although the Green Hill folks hadn't given us an eviction notice, it felt as if it were just around the corner.

It was inevitable that Mike would continue to lash out at other residents and caregivers. Also inevitable that sometime during such an incident, Elena or Livia, whomever was on the job, would realize she absolutely could no longer deal with Mike. Janell pointed out that the next desperate step would be for Elena/Livia to call 911 and tell them that Mike was beyond their capacity to control. He would be hospitalized. He would be frantic in the hospital. It would be impossible to reassure and calm him. He would have to be restrained. With both Green Hill and North Point closed to Mike, we would have no options for placement. The hospital would have to find the next place for him. It was sure to be a step down even from what North Point had to offer, and it would likely be in another county.

What a long, terrible, humiliating leave-taking Mike was suffering through.

THE OAK TREE POST-ACUTE CARE CENTER

2014

November. The Monday after the family Thanksgiving gathering at Dale and Marg's, Janell called to suggest that I visit the Oak Tree Post-Acute Care Center in Sacramento. She'd talked with the director who expressed a willingness to accept Mike. They had Medi-Cal beds available. Months earlier, having looked online at the Oak Tree's ratings, I'd crossed them off the list. Depending on who was doing the rating, CalGov, Yelp, or U. S. News & World Report, Oak Tree got either one or two stars out of a possible five. According to CalGov, the average time each patient got with nurses was well below the state average; the number of complaints was well above.

"Just take a look," Janell said. "They're under new management, with a new director. It might not be as bad as you think. It's probably better than wherever Mr. Reynolds would be placed in the event of a 911 call."

At Oak Tree I saw staff interacting with patients in a friendly and cheerful way. The halls were clean. It didn't smell bad. If I ignored the previous reviews, the Oak Tree met my now-minimal standards.

I described Mike's condition to the director, including his difficult behaviors and constant wandering. She glanced at an occupancy chart, said they had an open Medi-Cal bed, and we could move Mike in as soon as they received the necessary papers. Because we'd recently provided all of that information—recent medical evaluation, hospice records, notarized medical power of attorney, Physician Orders for Life-Sustaining Treatment, clear TB test results, etc., etc.—Janell had the completed packet at her fingertips. She faxed it in that afternoon, and we moved Mike to the Oak Tree the next day, December 9, 2014.

The first move to The Guiding Star at Porto Sicuro had included two boxes of framed pictures that the move organizers had hung on the wall before Mike arrived there. There was another box of picture albums, a single-sized extra long bed, a TV, a bedside table from our personal bedroom set, a favorite antique lamp, a full wardrobe of shirts, pants, pajamas, jackets, sweatshirts, shoes for all occasions, writing materials and a shelf of favorite books. With each following move, Mike's possessions had diminished, in keeping with his ongoing diminishing capacity to notice or make use of things. Where it had once taken two cars and a small truck to move Mike's possessions, the things we needed to take to the Oak Tree fit easily into the small trunk of the Prius. The list of items on the Oak Tree move-in form included five pair of pajamas, five shirts, and five pair of elastic waist sweat pants. The request for five each of those basic items was to allow for laundry turnaround. We also brought two pair of shoes and two framed family pictures. The pictures we hung on the wall at the foot of Mike's bed where, if he looked, he would see them upon awakening in the mornings. Everything fit into a narrow closet and the two drawers below the closet. There was a hospital-style curtain that divided Mike's space near the windows from his roommate's space near the door.

There was a large, secure, grassy area off the hall near where Mike's room was situated. Marg and I led him out there and watched as he looped around. It was much more spacious than the enclosed yard at Elena's, and Mike could make a complete loop there without backtracking. Maybe he could find a few anxiety-free moments circling the perimeter of the yard.

As far as Mike's adjustment to the new place, it hadn't seemed to make much difference to him one way or another. He walked the halls, looped through the outdoor space, took food from other patients' trays, picked up objects from other rooms and set them down elsewhere. He lashed out if anyone, staff or patient got in his way. After only a few hours there, the director called to say they found it necessary to bring in an extra caregiver exclusively for Mike.

The day after we moved Mike to Oak Tree, the director called and asked if I and a hospice representative could meet with her and the Oak Tree director of nursing the next afternoon. Once again, I relied on Marg's expertise to ease communications with the officials. In addition to Janell from hospice, the hospice doctor and director of nursing joined us. First on the agenda was the necessity of having individual 24-hour care for Mike until they could come up with a drug regimen that would calm him. They would bring in someone from their staff, but it would be at a fee of $20 an hour. This was certainly not an unreasonable cost. It probably meant that the caregiver would see $15 an hour of that at the most. The director of nursing said it could take a week or two, certainly not more than a month, to find the right balance of anti-anxiety, calming drugs. As soon as they found that balance, we could forgo the 24/7 extra care. While the hospice doctor and nurse, as well as the Oak Tree nurse, talked about possible drug regimens, I did the math. At $20 an hour, a day's care would cost $480. If it took a month to get Mike stabilized, that would be $14,480. Two weeks—$7,240. One week—$3,620. Even a week of such personalized care would cost more than a month at Elena's. So yes, Medi-Cal was covering the Oak Tree cost, but Medi-Cal would not cover the private 24/7 care.

"I can't do that," I said, interrupting the "which drug or combination of drugs might be most effective" conversation.

The Oak Tree director of nursing turned to me. "We can't manage Mr. Reynolds without that added care," she said.

At this point, Janell and the other hospice people began talking about possible ways to fund the added care. Janell spoke clearly and fervently on my behalf. Frankly, my head was spinning, and I don't remember the details, but ultimately, between some help from hospice and a hard-won agreement that the Oak Tree folks would provide the necessary added care for the next two weeks, I had dodged the $480-a-day bullet, at least for the moment.

After the rather grueling meeting, I went out into the hall to find Mike. He was making the rounds, his assigned caregiver right at his side. But before the caregiver could redirect him, Mike took a quick turn into a nearby room where an ancient-looking woman was propped up in her bed, eating lunch from a tray. Mike grabbed a glass of juice from the tray, and downed it before the caregiver could stop him.

"Help!" the woman screamed.

"Don't worry, sweetie, we'll get you another glass of juice," the caregiver reassured her.

"C'mon, Mike, let's see what the weather's like outside."

I led him to the outdoor area and walked with him, steering him away from the entrance back into the building each time he passed. It was a day of clear skies and weather in the high 60s. I breathed deeply of the crisp, clear air, relieved that, at least for now, things were okay for Mike at the Oak Tree.

We'd only been outside for a few minutes when the caregiver came out and stood next to me. He watched as Mike walked the perimeter. Smiling, he nodded toward Mike and said to me, "Too fast. Hard to keep up with."

"I know," I said. "He's especially fast when food is within reach."

This time when Mike reached the door to the hallway I didn't interfere.

"I'll be back tomorrow," I told the caregiver, who rushed to catch up with Mike.

I stopped for a minute to talk with the nurse for Mike's unit, telling her how much I appreciated their help.

"He's a tough one," she said. Then, smiling, she assured me, "Don't worry. We'll get him figured out."

I was again impressed with the gentle, good cheer the Oak Tree staff brought to their tasks.

We were in the middle of the Christmas season, a particularly poignant time, given the still fresh memories of Christmases with Mike—parties at our decorated-to-the-hilt Gold River house. Overnight visits from our kids and grandkids after our Christmas Eve dinners and opening of gifts, music, Christmas lasagna, eggnog, and Mike in the middle of it all, full of laughter and love. And although it had been a good, or not so good, six years since the Mike of laughter and love had been the instigator and energizer of our Christmas folderols, I still at times felt a fresh, fleeting stab of grief at the sound of a particular carol or the sight of an over-decorated tree. But Matt, Leesa, and Mika would soon be down from Walla Walla for our family celebration. We would gather at Sharon and Doug's, Lena and Subei's, in Woodacre. Dale, Marg, and Corry would join us, as would Cindi and family. It would be a happy time as new traditions gained purchase in our lives—heavier on happy than on sorrow.

After 10 days at the Oak Tree, Mike still needed his own individual caregiver 24/7, but it seemed things were going a little better. With each visit I was relieved to see that the staff seemed genuinely to like Mike. His roommate's wife found Mike to be troublesome because he often went after her husband's food, but she was not totally without empathy. Marg and I, along with Janell and other hospice staff, were scheduled to meet with the director again at the two-week point. I was sure we would be revisiting the issue of who was to pay for Mike's extra care, but the meeting was four days away, and I was in the "one day at a time" mode, enjoying pre-Christmas festivities.

On Friday evening, shortly after 9 o'clock, I'd been to dinner and a play with Dale and Marg and two other longtime friends. Driving home, still feeling buoyed by shared stories, laughter, and the ease of conversation that comes with longtime friends, my thoughts were interrupted by the jarring ring of my cell phone.

It was Robert, the night nurse on Mike's ward. He said Mike had started breathing heavily around 9 o'clock. He'd had his usual day, constantly walking the halls, taking food from other residents' trays, keeping the attendant assigned solely to him on his toes. He'd eaten three big meals along with whatever food he could find in between. Now his breathing pattern had changed. At first I didn't understand the significance of "breathing heavily."

"Should I come in the morning? Or now?"

"Now," Robert said, and I wondered about what could not be stated.

At the intersection I turned right toward the care center, rather than left toward home. I pulled to the side of the road long enough to select Dale's number on my cell phone, then continued on when the Bluetooth connection kicked in. Dale asked that I call back after I'd had chance to see what was going on.

I was parked in the Oak Tree lot by 9:30. The halls were dimly lit and, in contrast to the daytime bustle of attendants and nurses, visitors and patients, the place was eerily quiet. As I entered Mike's room, the LVN rose from her chair beside his bed and motioned for me to sit. Mike's eyes were open, but he didn't look my way when I entered the room nor did he show any recognition.

"Hi, Mike. I'm here," I said, leaning in close in front of his gaze.

It was obvious that his task was simply to breath— deep breath in, slight pause, breathe out, deep breath in, slight pause, breathe out. Although his breathing was labored, he did not seem distraught. I pulled the chair close to his bedside and stroked his thin-skinned, bony arm. Was he dying?

There had been several times over the past three, maybe four, years when one or another of the people who loved Mike would say they didn't think his body could keep going much longer, but keep going it did. Walking day and night. Eating day and night. Staying strong in spite of weight loss, chronic diarrhea, and eating nonfood items. For Mike's sake, and mine, for the sake of everyone who loved him, I'd long been wishing for Mike's body to give up—for Mike to be released from the horrible prison of extreme dementia. Now, paying attention to his every breath, I wondered if death might be imminent.

I told him I loved him. I thanked him for so many good times together, for our partnership in being mom and dad to Sharon, Cindi and Matt, our partnership in life. I thanked him for loving me.

How long had it been, I wondered, since Mike stayed in one place long enough for me to sit beside him and express any of my thoughts or feelings? But now, here he was, staying in one place, breathing in, breathing out. I felt his cool, skeletal forehead. I stroked his sunken cheek. I watched him breathe. I watched the steady pulse of a large vein in the crook of his left elbow. I remembered from the old days, the comfort of falling asleep with my head resting on his chest, lulled by the strong, unvarying beat of his heart.

After 15 minutes or so, I went out into the hall and called Matt, then Sharon, then Dale, to tell them of the changes. Sharon and Matt were often not immediately available by phone, but this time they were, and I was glad for that, though there was not much I could say, nothing they could do. I returned to Mike's room.

The room was an institutional grey, clean, smelling not of filth, but not of home. The over-bed rolling tray table sat against the wall next to the privacy curtain. There were several large plastic cups with tops, straws still inserted in some. A number of empty bowls and small plates took up the rest of the tray space. To a casual observer the contents of the tray would indicate dishes accumulated since breakfast or before, but I knew better. Mike, with his voracious appetite, his animal hunger, had emptied the contents of the plates, bowls and cups three or so hours earlier, at dinnertime.

I watched his breath, his pulse, and repositioned the light sheet over his pajama-clad emaciated body. I stood and leaned in, putting my face in front of what appeared to be his pathway of vision. The focus of his eyes did not change. His breathing had become slightly more labored.

The LVN came in to ask if I'd like water, or tea. I told her no, thank you, but that I appreciated the offer. She smiled, then quietly rolled the over-bed tray out and down the hall. Robert came in to check on Mike, stood and watched, took his pulse. I followed him out of the room and asked what he thought. He repeated what he'd told me over the phone. Mike ate a lot during the day. He walked the halls continuously. After dinner, Mike got into bed of his own accord—a first. Something had changed. Robert didn't know what. The pattern of Mike's breathing had changed. Robert didn't think Mike was in pain. I hoped that was true. It seemed as if it were true.

I went back to the chair by Mike's bedside. He was breathing harder. I wondered if his body was giving up. For so many years I'd wondered how much longer he could go on, and he'd kept going on. Now I watched his pulse. I listened to him breathe. I told him again that I loved him. I thanked him again for all of the good times. I rested my hand against his dry bony cheek.

"I'm okay," I said. "These have been some hard, hard years, but I'm okay. It's okay for you to let go."

I told him this just in case there remained within him a sliver of understanding.

I watched each breath. I listened as his struggle grew stronger. I watched his pulse.

Sometime after 10 his breathing became less regular, with occasional pauses between breaths. A while later a soft rattle came with intermittent breaths. The pulse in his arm beat on. His work was harder now, the pauses longer. By 10:30 some of the pauses were so long I wondered if he'd taken his final breath. I repeated what had now become a mantra: *I love you. Thank you for so many good times. Thank you for loving me. Thank you for being a good dad. It's okay to let go.*

Around 10:45 there was a very long pause in Mike's breath. The pulse in his arm was no longer visible. I pressed my fingers to that place in the crook of his arm. Nothing. The pulse place in his neck. Nothing. He made a deep gasp, then quiet. I sat watching. Waiting. It was as if I were looking down on the scene from a great distance. I saw Mike stretched out and silent. I saw me sitting close beside him. All at a distance.

It was close to 11 when Dale and Marg came into the room. I stood to greet them. "He's gone," I said.

Mike gasped another inhale.

Marg went to his side, touched him. Kissed his forehead. Felt for a pulse. We watched and waited. Was there one more gasp? I thought so, though I wasn't sure. Did Marg close Mike's eyes? I'm not sure of that either. The LVN came in and offered to clean Mike up. Marg said that would be nice and we left the room. After a while the nurse came out with a bundle of dirty laundry, and we went back to Mike's bed. His face looked more relaxed and peaceful than I'd seen it in years.

"Do you want some time alone with him?" Marg asked.

"I had that before you got here," I said, and went back out into the hallway.

For the past few years, ever since Mike was no longer Mike, I'd been wishing for his body to let him go. My wish finally fulfilled, it seemed almost too much to take in. As I went through the motions of dealing with details, I felt as if I were seeing everything, myself included, from a distance—functioning while floating suspended in limbo.

I called Matt, then Sharon. We said what people say: *It's sad. It was time. He's finally free. They wished they could have been here. I wished so, too, and reminded them that they had been constant supports despite geographical distances.*

I called Cindi. She, too, expressed a mix of sadness and relief. There were more phone calls to be made, but there was no need to interrupt people's sleep. This news could wait until morning.

I called the University of California, San Francisco, Memory and Aging Center to confirm the prearranged plan for the donation of Mike's brain. But because Mike died on a Friday, things were more complicated than they would have been on a weekday. There would be no one at UCSF to receive his body until Monday. Nautilus would have to transport his body to a local mortuary, where it would be stored until Monday. Then Nautilus would again have to transport Mike's body to UCSF. The Nautilus contract covered transportation from the place of death to a place of cremation. They would cover transport to the local mortuary, but the trip to UCSF, then the trip from UCSF to a crematorium would be extra. There would, of course, be a daily fee for mortuary storage. I chose to forgo the brain donation.

In hindsight, I wish I'd stayed with the donation plan because FTD research is so needed. I wish I'd figured out that I could manage the $500 or so added costs. But I had to make a quick decision one way or the other. And I was so used to having absolutely no discretionary funds that I couldn't see my way clear to say yes to another big expense. So Nautilus transported Mike's body straight to the local crematorium.

A week later UPS delivered the cremains, the outside of the package clearly labeled, in red, "Contains Human Cremains." Inside the package was a heavy bag that contained a securely fastened, sturdy plastic box, again with the "Human Cremains" label, plus Mike's full name, Social Security number, and dates of birth and death.

I placed the package on a high shelf in the garage. Sometime later, I and the rest of the family would come up with a plan for dispersal. In the meantime, there were many other things to attend to—sending death notices to the California State Teachers' Retirement System, to Social Security, and to an insurance company where Mike had maintained a small, paid-up policy. Getting multiple copies of our marriage certificate to include with the death certificates. Providing proper documents to the credit union that would allow them to remove his name from a joint account. Cancel Mike's health insurance policy. Etc., etc., etc.

We gathered for Christmas only six days after Mike's death. Scattered throughout the frivolity of that year's celebration, and the extreme levity that Dale's 70th birthday prompted, were remembrances of Mike, expressions of our collective and individual grief, and a recognition of our shared relief that his long and torturous ordeal was over.

February 2016

Dear Mike,

Awake at 4 this morning, I took my iPad from the bedside table and tapped it on. Up came Our Souls at Night *by Kent Haruf, published posthumously. I'd pre-ordered the e-book in January and have been waiting for it with a combination of eager impatience and foreboding. Books published after an author's death always worry me. What if the book wasn't ready yet? What if putting it out into the world was simply a business decision made by the author's publisher and family?*

I may not even read Go Set a Watchman, *the novel Harper Lee wrote in the '50s, before she wrote* To Kill A Mockingbird, *and which is just now being published. Ms. Lee has been adamant over the years that she would not write or release another novel. Now that she's 89, in assisted living, without oversight by her recently deceased sister and caregiver, the old manuscript has suddenly been rediscovered. Of course, it will be a huge moneymaker, but Ms. Lee is in no need of money. Someone else may be, though. I'm afraid to read it. On the other hand, if it's only half as good as* To Kill a Mockingbird, *it will be well worth the read.*

But the impetus for this letter is Our Souls at Night, *Kent Haruf's recently released novel and my early morning reading and ruminations, not the pitfalls of posthumous publishing. Although I'm determined to live in the present, plan for the near future, and trust the farther future to the forces of the universe, I'm often drawn back to our lives together, especially those last most difficult years, especially in the silence of the very early morning hours.*

This early morning, I read Kent Haruf's depiction of two old people—a man and a woman—who had recently become close companions, and were sharing stories of their earlier lives. The man, Louis, is telling Addie about the moment of his wife's death. He and his daughter, Holly, were in the room with her:

"She stared at us with those big dark eyes like she was saying, 'Help me. Help me. Why won't you help me?' Then she quit breathing and was gone. People say the spirit stays around for a while floating over the body and maybe hers did. Holly said she had the sense of her mother being in the room and maybe I did too. I couldn't be sure. I felt something. Some kind of emanation. But it was very slight, maybe just a breath. I don't know. At least she's at peace now in some other place or higher realm. I think

I believe that. I hope she is."

The passage caused me to wonder if I'd left your bedside too soon after your final breath, if your spirit had hovered, seeking me while I, ever practical, was at the nurses' station calling Nautilus. If so, I'm sorry. I'm sorry for that, and for so much more, though I do at least take comfort in having been with you during your last hours, and telling you things which, because of your constant movement, I'd not been able to tell you for years. And I take comfort that I was by your side, my hand on your arm, as you breathed your last.

Now, more than a year later, Kent Haruf's character has raised the possibility that the spirit stays around for a while floating over the body, and I wonder if that was the case for you, if you were looking for me, and I wasn't there. I'm reminded of how, in the early stages of FTD, before I had any idea of what was going on with your brain, you would call me on my cell phone, sounding angry, saying, "I don't know where you are!" And I would tell you, the store, the gym, the writing group, and then, just minutes later you would call again: "I don't know where you are!"

Once I came home from the market to find you pacing in front of the garage. "I couldn't find you!"

I was always careful to tell you where I was going and when I would be back, and your rude, angry phone calls when I was away angered me. Now I know that no matter what I'd told you, or what notes I'd left on the refrigerator, you had lost the capacity to know where I was. Now I think your anger must have been based in fear. And now I wish I had stayed by your hospital bed longer, in case your spirit was trying to find me.

Marilyn

GATHERING
January 10, 2015

FTD had started chipping away at the essence of Mike some time in 2005, and by the time of his death in 2014, the image of the emaciated, lashing out, constantly walking shell of Mike had essentially overpowered memories of better times. Yes, there would be times when a song or an anecdote would remind me of the Mike I'd married, my close life-partner for the pre-FTD 38 years of our marriage. But for the last six years of his life, nearly all of my psychic space was filled with witnessing Mike's decline, managing his care, struggling to keep him from being evicted from first one place and then another, fruitlessly trying to find a calming drug or behavior technique that would keep him from being a danger to those around him, and through it all I was watching helplessly as all semblances of financial security slipped into oblivion.

As is true for most of my contemporaries, communication through social media doesn't seem quite right to me. Because of my work as a writer, though, I'd followed the advice of another writer friend and set up a Facebook account. This was several years earlier. I can't say that it helped sell books, but I did find it to be a treasure when it came to reconnecting with long ago friends. So I posted Mike's obituary on Facebook. Within hours, former students were posting tributes to him. He was the reason one now teaches music. Another is singing professionally. He was the only one she could turn to when, at the age of 16, she realized she was pregnant. His class was all that kept another student coming to school. And on and on, such touching tributes not only from former students, but from others who had sung with Mike, or under his direction. Several spoke of his many kindnesses. All reminders of the Mike who had faded from memory.

We organized a memorial service for January 10, so Subei could be a part of it before she went back to college in Ohio. Mike's Florida niece, Beth, arrived on the Thursday before the Saturday service. The other out-of-towners came in on Friday. I'd invited anyone who wanted to sleep on the floor to stay at my place (no one took me up on that), and directed the others to a nearby "unfussy all-suite hotel." I'd also invited the out-of-towners and other close friends and family to my place for drinks and appetizers that Friday evening. Left to my own devices, appetizers and drinks would likely have been hummus and spinach dip with pita chips and a few bottles of Two-Buck-Chuck in each color. But luckily for all in attendance, I wasn't left to my own devices.

Sharon came in early to help, bringing with her multiple bottles of wine that promised not to offend the palates of my more discerning guests. She also brought with her some fancy cheeses and artisanal crackers. She and Beth did a run to the market while I gave the duplex the kind of cleanup job my mother would have referred to as "a lick and a promise."

In my *Art of Entertaining* manual, the page of instructions for how to make things look pretty on a plate must be missing. I knew which cupboard held the pretty plates, but beyond that I was useless in the "make pretty" department. In my previous life, Mike had made things pretty while I took care of practicalities. Now it was up to Sharon to carry on in her father's tradition. By 4 in the afternoon, when our first out-of-towner, Bill Schmidt, arrived, there was a vast array of appetizers beautifully displayed on the kitchen/living room bar, and acceptable wine ready to pour into Mike's crystal glasses.

Soon there were more people crowded into my little duplex than it had likely ever seen before at one time. Kids and grandkids, longtime Southern California friends, people Mike had sung with, or taught with, or traveled with, told sweet, funny, quintessentially Mike stories. Most of the people in the room had experienced puzzling, at times hurtful, behavior as FTD was gaining a foothold, but other than close family, none had witnessed the anxiety-ridden, enraged, uncomprehending, combative version of the Mike that had filled my waking and sleeping life for the previous five to six years. Now, though, in this place filled with love of Mike, and of each other, pieces of pre-FTD memories pushed through the heavy dark clouds of the recent past, and the whole of the man I'd loved and lived with rose toward the surface of my consciousness, waiting to be restored.

JUST THE FACTS

Every drug listed is one Mike took during the course of the designated year. Due to gaps in my records, start and stop dates are not often listed, nor are dosage changes.

Attempts to treat Mike's depression/anxiety through drugs often brought a positive change for a short period of time, though sometimes it took a week or so to see any effects. The positive change might last for just a few days up to a month or so, then Mike's level of depression/anxiety would return to a pre-drug treatment level, as if he had a set point that was stronger than any medication could counteract.

2005

BEHAVIORS:
- Panic attack at choral concert.
- It seemed that times of indifference and a general disinterest in me were becoming more frequent, though that was hard to measure. This wasn't totally new behavior, but my sense was that the frequency of such behavior had increased. Generally, the changes were subtle and nothing others were noticing.

PRESCRIPTION DRUGS:
- Zocor (simvastatin), 40 mg. Cholesterol-lowering drug. One of the more serious side effects is confusion and memory problems, though I wasn't aware of that at this time.
- Zoloft (sertraline), 50 mg. An antidepressant of the selective serotonin reuptake inhibitor (SSRI) class.

2006

BEHAVIORS:
- Indifference, disinterest more the norm. Increased dissatisfaction with all things Sacramento. Increased dissatisfaction with UUSS Music Director position. Ranting about politics, the behavior of others, whatever irritated him. Calm discussion was not often possible. Stopped regular exercise. Began weight gain.

PRESCRIPTION DRUGS:

- Cymbalta (duloxetine), 30 mg. to 60 mg. For treatment of major depressive disorder and/or generalized anxiety disorder. The only side effect that might have been at play at this time would be agitation.
- Wellbutrin (bupropion), 150 mg. (started 9/14/06, stopped 4/23/07). Antidepressant. May be add-on in cases of incomplete response to SSRI. May impair thinking or reactions.
- Zocor (simvastatin), 40 mg. Cholesterol-lowering drug.
- Zoloft (sertraline), 50 mg. Antidepressant.

2007

BEHAVIORS:

- Continued increase of indifference and self-absorption with me.
- Occasional indifference and self-absorption now exhibited with others. Continued increase in dissatisfaction with life: Sacramento, loss of Yip Harburg project, need to conform to HOA's requirements. Lessened ability to understand or accept the opinions of others. Increasing frequency of ranting. Incapacity to focus on positive aspects of life for even 15 minutes. Occasional difficulty keeping track of appointments or social engagements. Longer time periods of depression with increased severity.

PRESCRIPTION DRUGS:

- Cymbalta (duloxetine), 30 mg. to 60 mg. For treatment of major depressive disorder and/or generalized anxiety disorder.
- Lipitor (atorvastatin), 80 mg. (started 4/08/08). Drug class of statins. Cholesterol-lowering drug.
- Topamax (topiramate), 25 gm. (started 9/26/07). Anticonvulsant. Sometimes used to treat bipolar disorder, borderline personality disorder, may have mood-stabilizing properties. (As of May 21, 2010, there was no data from any well-controlled clinical trial to show that Topamax was safe and/or effective to treat any psychiatric conditions.)
- Vytorin (ezetimibe/simvastatin), 10 mg. of one drug, 80 mg. of another, lipid-lowering drug.

- Wellbutrin (buproprion), 150 mg. (started 9/14/06, stopped 4/23/07). Antidepressant.
- Zocor (simvastatin), 40 mg. (stopped 4/23/07). Cholesterol-lowering drug. One of the more serious side effects is confusion, memory problems.

2008

BEHAVIORS/EVENTS:

- More pronounced indifference and self-absorption, including with others. Continued increase in free-floating dissatisfaction with life: Sacramento, my schedule, church choir details. Growing inability to understand or accept the opinions of others. Often self-centered. "Conversation" consists mainly of ranting. Unwillingness to focus on positive aspects of life. Growing difficulty keeping track of appointments or social engagements. Continued depression with increased severity. Complaints of headaches and generally feeling unwell. Calling Sharon in the middle of her busy workday, sometimes saying, "I don't know where Mom is," and wanting to talk at length.
- Repeating the same stories as if stuck on them—how unpredictable his mother was, how he hated the squirrels that he thought were scaring the humming-birds, how racist his younger brother was, etc.
- No longer able to use ATM.

PRESCRIPTION DRUGS:
(Ongoing unless otherwise noted. 1 per day unless otherwise noted.):
- ASA (acetylsalicylic acid, or aspirin), 81 mg.
- Cymbalta (duloxetine), 60 mg. twice daily. For treatment of major depressive disorder and/or generalized anxiety disorder. The only side effect that might possibly have been at play at this time would be agitation.
- Ritalin (methylphenidate), 5 mg. For suspected AD/HD
- Topamax (topiramate), 25 mg. Anticonvulsant. Sometimes used to treat bipolar disorder, borderline personality disorder, may have mood-stabilizing properties.
- Zetia (ezetimibe), 10 mg. Cholesterol-lowering drug.

2009

BEHAVIORS/EVENTS:

- Self-centered, emotionally withdrawn, often unaware of others' emotions.
- Outbursts of frustration, diminished social tact.
- Difficulty reasoning, poor judgment, can't keep track of appointments or organize music.
- So anxious about getting places on time, may show up an hour or more early, then leave, angry that what he expects to happen isn't happening.
- Watches same movies repeatedly, constant repetition of phrases and stories, "I never walk out of a movie," "They called me Mikey when I was a boy," etc.
- Constant use of washing machine and dishwasher with very small loads.
- Increasing trouble naming people, objects, facts and words.
- Speech keeps regular speed and rhythm but filled with inaccuracies.
- Can no longer function as choral director for Chanteuses.
- Mandatory "medical leave" from Westminster Presbyterian Church.

PRESCRIPTION DRUGS:

- Xanax (alprazolam), .5 mg. Generalized anxiety disorder, panic disorder.
- Cerefolin-NAC. Prescription-strength vitamin supplement.
- Concerta (methylphenidate), 27 mg. For suspected AD/HD.
- Cymbalta (duloxetine), 60mg. Major depressive disorder, generalized anxiety.
- Erythromycin Base, 250 mg. Antibiotic.
- Lunesta (eszopiclone), 3 mg. Insomnia.
- Namenda (memantine HCI), 10 mg. Alzheimer's, though sometimes used for other dementias.
- Trazodone, 50 mg. Antidepressant.
- Zetia (ezetimibe), 10 mg. Cholesterol-lowering drug.

2010

BEHAVIORS/EVENTS:

- Consistently self-centered, emotionally withdrawn, unaware of others' emotions.
- Increased outbursts of frustration, severely diminished social tact.

- Difficulty reasoning, poor judgment, can't keep track of appointments or organize music, has lost the ability to understand time sequences. Telling him we'd do something later in the day, or tomorrow, or the next week, was the same thing as telling him we would be doing it right now.
- No longer licensed to drive.
- Rather than showing up an hour early for an event, he now feels a strong need to go days earlier than scheduled.
- Watches same movies repeatedly, though will often not be able to accurately state what he's been watching. For example, after seeing "Singin' in the Rain," looping from morning to afternoon one day, I asked what he'd been watching. "Moulin Rouge" was his answer.
- Although still repeating certain phrases and stories, he hardly ever initiates conversation.
- Increasing trouble naming people, objects, facts and words.
- Speech continues to keep regular speed and rhythm but is mostly inaccurate.
- Sometimes refuses to shower, wants to wear same clothes day after day.
- Continues to capably play the piano.
- December 10, 2010, moved to secure memory care facility.

PRESCRIPTION DRUGS:
- Lipitor (arovastatin), 10 mg. Cholesterol-lowering drug.
- Cymbalta (duloxetine), 60 mg. Major depressive disorder, generalized anxiety.
- Ritalin ER (methylphenidate), 27 mg. AD/HD.
- Namenda (memantine), 10 mg. Alzheimer's, though sometimes used for other dementias.
- Risperdal (risperidone), 0.5 mg. Anti-psychotic.
- Flomax (tamsulosin), 0.4 mg. For ease of urination in men with enlarged prostate.

2011

BEHAVIORS/EVENTS:
- Less able/willing to shave or cut fingernails.
- Unsociable at The Guiding Star facility dining room.
- Lashes out at caregivers.

- Intermittently incontinent.
- Intermittent bouts of diarrhea.
- Regularly tries to "escape" from The Guiding Star.
- Plays the piano less often and less well.
- Other than, "Let's go," when I visit, his capacity for self-expression is quite limited. Gives short, often inaccurate, answers to questions.
- Often yells, "Fuck you!" at caregivers and fellow residents.

PRESCRIPTION DRUGS:
- Depakote (divalproex sodium), 500 mg. For agitation and aggression. An anti-convulsant and mood stabilizer. It suppresses the spread of abnormal electrical discharges, relieving the symptoms of disorders such as epilepsy, bipolar disorder, and migraine headaches. Side effects may include drowsiness, diarrhea, nausea and/or vomiting, fatigue/weakness, tremor, headache, asthenia, indigestion, stomach cramps, slurred speech, insomnia, nervousness, respiratory infection, blurred vision, flu syndrome, liver irritation, pancreas problems, weight gain, ringing or buzzing of the ears, hallucinations/psychosis, sedation, tremor, dizziness, abdominal pain, rash, hair loss.
- Lipitor (atorvastin), 80 mg. (started 4/08/08). Drug class of statins. Cholesterol-lowering drug.
- Namenda (memantine), 10 mg. Alzheimer's, though sometimes used for other dementias.
- Trazodone, 50 mg. Antidepressant.
- Zyprexa (olanzapine), 2.5 mg. An atypical antipsychotic. Approved for treatment of schizophrenia and bipolar disorder.

2012

BEHAVIORS/EVENTS:
- Often needs help getting dressed.
- Bouts of diarrhea are more frequent. Lab tests, blood panel, and stool samples show no apparent cause.
- Needs more help with showers and shaving.
- Increased blankness in affect.
- Mostly one- or two-word answers to direct questions with random accuracy.

- Increasingly agitated and violent at The Guiding Star.
- Arrested early February for violent, out-of-control behavior.
- Moved to Sister Sarah's.
- Constantly walking a loop around and through the house at Sister Sarah's.
- Totally incontinent.
- Persistent twitching of Mike's right wrist when walking or standing.
- Sang cuts drug intake to include just one anti-anxiety drug, Seroquel (quetiapine fumarate).
- Lashes out at residents who get in his way.
- Takes food from other residents.
- Often removes shirt and shoes.
- Eats constantly and voraciously.
- Steady weight loss.
- Occasionally walks bent and crooked, leaning to his right at an extreme angle.

*PRESCRIPTION DRUGS:
- Lipitor (atorvastatin), 80 mg. Statin. Cholesterol-lowering drug.
- Celexa, (citalopram), 20 mg. Anxiety and agitation.
- Depakote (divalproex sodium), 500 mg. Agitation and aggression.
- HCA Aspirin, 81 mg. Heart health.
- Zyprexa (olanzapine), 5 mg., severe dementia agitation and aggression
- Miralax (polyethylene glycol 3350, 71 gr. Anti-diarrhea.
- Seroquel (quetiapine fumarate), 300 mg. Atypical antipsychotic, approved for schizophrenia, bipolar disorder.
- Trazodone, 50 mg. Stated use now for agitation and insomnia. Previously prescribed for depression.

*By the end of 2012, Sang had weaned Mike off all drugs except for Seroquel.

2013

BEHAVIORS/EVENTS:
- Mike receives Medi-Cal approval as a potential Assisted Living Waiver resident.
- In September, Sister Sarah's gives a 30-day notice of eviction. Motivation is unclear.

- Move to Green Hill Care Home, another six-bed residential facility.
- Weight now down from 190 pounds when he entered Sister Sarah's to 160 pounds on entry to Green Hill.
- Near miss for move to Assisted Living Waiver facility.
- Cutting fingernails and toenails is an extremely difficult three-person job.
- Continued "looping," but with more limited outdoor space.
- A series of Green Hill caregivers quit because of Mike's violent behavior.
- Broken teeth, abscessed gum.
- Complicated and largely unsatisfactory dental care.
- Continued voracious eating. Continued, consistent weight loss.
- Only speech is in one-word answers to simple, direct questions.
- No longer initiates any speech, even "hello," or "hi."

PRESCRIPTION DRUGS:
- Seroquel (quetiapine fumarate), 300 mg. Atypical antipsychotic, approved for schizophrenia, bipolar disorder

2014

BEHAVIORS/EVENTS:
- As a result of Mike's ongoing weight loss and a "failure to thrive," Mike qualifies for hospice care, which offers invaluable support, both emotionally and in practical matters.
- Often seems not to recognize family visitors.
- Continued lashing out. Other residents fearful of Mike. Their family members are concerned.
- Mike's ravenous appetite results in attempts to consume inedible items such as puzzle pieces, the foam from a resident's safety helmet, etc.
- On a visit to Mike on a hot July day, I discover that he is locked outside.
- After a 90-day evaluation, Mike is dropped from hospice care.
- Elena and Livia seem more and more stressed over the difficulties of caring for Mike. I fear another 30-day eviction notice.
- Early September. Mike falls, hits his head on the floor, gets up and continues walking.

- His head is bleeding. Livia is unable to get a close enough look to assess the extent of the injury. Calls 911. Mike is taken to the emergency hospital. Turns out to be a minor injury.
- Mike again qualifies for hospice care. The hospice social worker helps renew the search for a Medi-Cal facility. One after another, local facilities turn down our applications because of Mike's behavior until, finally, he is accepted by the Oak Tree Post-Acute Care Center in Sacramento.
- Move to Oak Tree on December 9.
- December 19, 9 p.m. The night nurse calls to say that Mike has started breathing heavily. I am at his bedside by 9:30. A little after 11, Mike breathes his last. Finally released from the bonds of frontotemporal dementia.

PRESCRIPTION DRUGS:
- Until December, no drugs except for occasional use of Valium for dental examinations.
- December 9, entry to Oak Tree. Mike received something for sedation, anxiety, agitation, though I'm unsure of the specific drugs.

WHERE TO FIND HELP

Below is just a scattering of possibilities for help and support for people who are, in one way or another, dealing with FTD, or other forms of dementia. In general, if you can connect with a local social worker or RN, they can save you a lot of time in your search for help. Your medical provider can steer you to other areas of help.

The Association for Frontotemporal Degeneration (AFTD),
http://www.theaftd.org

This website offers a wealth of information, including how to find support groups, managing health care and legal and financial planning, etc., etc. It also offers ways to get involved in the organization, reports on research, related news reports, and more. I highly recommend *The Doctor Thinks It's FTD. Now What? A Guide for Managing a New Diagnosis.* It can be found under the "Life with FTD" tab. It offers much needed information and guidance. Published in 2013, it's exactly what I and others who loved Mike needed in 2009.

Alzheimer's Association, http://www.alz.org

As with AFTD, this organization offers help on all aspects of dealing with dementia. Although Alzheimer's and FTD differ in the way the diseases attack the brain, symptoms often overlap. In some areas, Alzheimer's support groups are more prolific than are FTD support groups. Any dementia support group, whether or not it's labeled FTD, can be helpful.

HOSPICE CARE SERVICES

Hospice agencies vary from area to area. Your doctor or medical group will be able to refer you to an appropriate service. Even if the person you're caring for seems not to fit hospice criteria, it's worth discussing such possibilities with your medical provider. I was surprised when Mike qualified for hospice care, but once set up, hospice significantly eased our way.

Based on previous experiences as a hospice nurse, Marg had a strong preference for a nonprofit service. Our first hospice experience with Mike was with a nonprofit. They were extremely supportive in practical matters, securing a hospital bed, providing twice-weekly LVN visits that helped with matters of hygiene and general care, and keeping check on Mike physically. They also offered invaluable emotional support. On the second and final round with hospice, we had a for-profit service. Their services were equally caring and competent.

IN-HOME CARE

Again these services vary from area to area. Both the AFTD and Alzheimer's Association can offer basic guidelines. Depending on where you live, financial aid for in home care may be available through the Health and Human Services agency that serves your state.

COMMUNITY SENIOR CENTERS

Tax assistance, legal hotlines, adult day care programs, these centers usually offer referrals to a host of free or low cost, trustworthy community resources.

Del Oro Caregiver Resource Center, http://www.deloro.org.
This is a nonprofit organization that provides a variety of no-cost services to residents of 13 Northern California counties. Their services include counseling, respite care, legal/financial consultations, and education and training related to caregiving. Their help was invaluable to me both emotionally and in practical matters of negotiating the bankruptcy maze.

PRIVATE REFERRAL SERVICES FOR RESIDENTIAL CARE

Senior Care Solutions, http://www.seniorcs.com
Carol Kinsel of Senior Care Solutions was a great help and support throughout the nearly six years of this most difficult journey with my FTD-afflicted husband. Senior Care generally serves the greater Sacramento area, but they are also knowledgeable about similar services in other areas.

Senior Care Solutions offers monthly talks/discussions with experts on various aspects of caregiving, i.e., veteran's benefits, caring as a family, dealing with grief, etc. Each of these meetings that I've attended has been excellent.

The Internet offers listings for senior placement services in the greater United States. My experience has been that word-of-mouth referrals are most helpful in finding trustworthy services, but sometimes the Internet provides a good start.

FOR MEDICAL DIAGNOSES
UCSF Department of Neurology, Memory and Aging Center
http://memory.ucsf.edu

Mayo Clinic Department of Neurology, **http://www.mayoclinic.org/ departments-centers/neurology/home/**

Specifically for frontotemporal dementia, http://www.mayoclinic. org/diseases-conditions/frontotemporal-dementia/basics/definition/ con-20023876

Most teaching hospitals have departments of neurology. You can find teaching hospitals in your state at: **http://www.ushospital.info/teaching.htm**

FOR THE SAKE OF SCIENCE
You can get information on clinical trials at:
https://www.google.com/search?client=safari&rls=en&q=clinical+trials+for +frontotemporal+dementia&ie=UTF-8&oe=UTF-8

Brain donation, specifically FTD:
http://www.theaftd.org/life-with-ftd/participate-in-research/brain-donation

Brain donation, general information:
 https://neurobiobank.nih.gov/pages/donor/

FOR THE SAKE OF YOUR OWN SANITY

According to some sources, 60 percent of caregivers die before those they're caring for do. One study claims that caregiving extends the life expectancy of the caregiver. I seriously doubt that, but the 60 percent figure also seems high. What is known for certain, though, is that caregivers are more prone to depression. Their immune systems are compromised. They tend to neglect their own health needs. Exercise habits fall by the wayside. Needs for personal time go unmet. How to balance the needs of the declining person you love with your own needs? There are no easy answers to that one, and what's helpful to one won't be to another. But here are a few things that I, or others, found to ease our way.

Friends and family! Independent to a fault, I found it difficult asking for and accepting help. But I got over that. Many of our circle truly wanted to help. And I truly needed help. The lunches, movies, and various outings with Mike that others provided gave me some much-needed breathing space. A chance to read, to write, to dawdle at the computer, to meet a friend for coffee, such times offered nourishing renewal for my depleted spirit.

These folks can also offer important reality checks. Although looking back on my husband's decline it doesn't seem that it was gradual. I adapted to his changes without always consciously registering them. It was the "frog in the soup pot" syndrome. Someone who knows you both but doesn't see your ward on a daily basis can more clearly see the extent of the changes he or she is exhibiting. Such an outside observer can help you avoid getting to the boiling point.

Support groups for dementia caregivers and other community resources. Both the national Association for Frontotemporal Degeneration (theaftd. org) and the Alzheimer's Association (alz.org) list support group resources available per region.

Churches, assisted living facilities, medical centers and senior centers also often offer support for caregivers.

Communication. It is easy to become so enmeshed in the demands of caregiving that you lose touch with the outside world. Early on Mike took on toddler behavior and demanded attention whenever I was engaged in telephone conversations. For me at that time, email became my lifeline.

Mike had a wide circle of concerned friends, all wanting to know how he was doing. At first I tried to let all interested parties know by email but soon found that to be problematic. I might forget to include someone in a group email. Or I might say more in a group email than some would want to know. Shortly after his diagnosis, I started a "Friends of Mike's" blog, in which I posted updates every week or two. The last year or two of Mike's life, blog entries became less frequent, but the blog was, I know, helpful to some readers—maybe even more helpful to this writer.

Professional therapy or counseling. During the most difficult years, every two weeks or so, I met with the psychiatrist who had previously worked with Mike. It was helpful to talk with an "outsider" who had close-up knowledge of Mike and his condition, but who was not emotionally entangled. Our conversations often enabled me to think more deeply about the situation that I, and Mike, were in. I still see this doctor, though since Mike's death my visits are less frequent.

Exercise! Before caring for Mike became too confining, I'd consistently participated in a "sculpt and stretch" class at a local gym, and had also walk/jogged (mostly walked) on the gym treadmill three times a week. Out of necessity, I walked the dog three to four times a day, but these walks hardly qualified as exercise. When I moved Mike to a "facility," I again had more opportunity to exercise. By that time I could no longer afford gym membership, but more lengthy, vigorous walks helped. Both mood and energy level greatly improved with exercise.

Something that feeds your soul. For me that was friends and family, reading, working on writing projects, and working with at-risk teen readers/writers. During the time that Mike was needing major attention, I occasionally worked with local incarcerated youth in a writing program. I also managed time for a few author visits to high schools. I worked sporadically on a collection of personal essays. *Over 70 and I Don't Mean MPH: Reflections on the Gift of Longevity* (2012) was a mostly lighthearted look at the joys and challenges of aging. I'd originally thought the 70+ book would include stories of Mike's dementia, and of my taking care of him, but the balance was off, hence the book you are now reading. During most of this time I managed to participate in a weekly writing group—another opportunity for much-needed renewal.

For my whole life, at least since the first Nancy Drew mystery I read sometime around the age of 7 or 8, reading has been a source of entertainment, a connection to the wider world, intellectual and spiritual growth, and, sometimes, healing. From about 2007, maybe 2008, most of my reading time was when Mike was sleeping. I had one of those tiny booklights and, if I turned away from him, was able to read in the late-night/early-morning hours. Unlike a lot of serious readers, I don't record what I've read, so the following book list is incomplete. But here are some that I found to be helpful during this very hard time of life:

BOOKS THAT EASED MY WAY (A PARTIAL LIST)

Strange Relation: A Memoir of Marriage, Dementia, and Poetry, Rachel Hadas. This was one of those books that shows up when one most needs it. It was probably spring of 2011, shortly after it was published, when I first found it. I was lonely for the husband I'd once known, feeling guilty that I either couldn't or wouldn't care for him on my own, frustrated that, even with Mike in residential care, the demands of watching out for him, plus living with financial disaster, were keeping me from any concerted writing time. More than anything Rachel Hadas' story let me know that I was not alone. She is a poet and scholar. Her husband was a musician. It seemed we had some things in common. She, too, was puzzled by her husband's changes in behavior. By his lack of concern for her. Guilt. Frustration. Demands on her time. Loneliness. There were so many parallels in our experiences, it was as if we were sharing a lifeboat—so much easier to row with two people handling the oars rather than handling them solo.

The Theft of Memory: Losing My Father, One Day at a Time, Jonathan Kozol. Kozol's father, a neurologist and psychiatrist, was diagnosed with Alzheimer's in 1994 and died in 2008. A touching account of a son's struggle to maintain contact with his beloved, declining father.

Dancing Fish and Ammonites, Penelope Lively. In-depth reflections on aging.

Are You in a Caregiving Relationship and Don't Know it? Finding the Balance of Loving and Caring, Wendy Packer and Linda J. Parker. Emphasizes importance of caring for one's self while caring for others.

What If It's Not Alzheimer's? A Caregiver's Guide to Dementia, Gary Radin and Lisa Radin. The only book we could find back in 2009 that dealt specifically with FTD. Offers important practical advice and a thorough list of resources.

To Love What Is: A Marriage Transformed, Alix Kate Shulman. Shulman's husband suffers a traumatic brain injury, forever changing their lives. This beautifully written memoir tells the story of how she copes with the changes and continues to love her diminished husband.

A Three Dog Life, Abigail Thomas. After a tragic accident that leaves her husband so severely brain damaged that he must be institutionalized, Thomas struggles to maintain a relationship with the man who still offers glimpses of his old, loving self. She also struggles to build a new life.

The Other Side of Sadness: What the New Science of Bereavement Tells Us About Life After Loss, George A. Bonanno. This offers a more complex, and ultimately more positive, look at the grieving process than our simplistic understanding of grief as a rigid five-step process.

The 36-Hour Day: A Family Guide to Caring for People Who Have Alzheimer Disease, Related Dementias, and Memory Loss, Nancy L. Mace and Peter V. Rabins

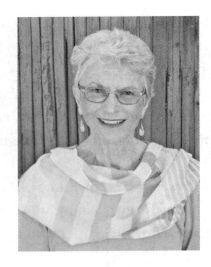

Marilyn Reynolds is the author of 10 books of realistic teen fiction in the "True-to-Life Series from Hamilton High," a book for educators, *I Won't Read and You Can't Make Me: Reaching Reluctant Teen Readers,* and a collection of personal essays, *Over 70 and I Don't Mean MPH.* She started work on *'Til Death or Dementia Do Us Part* shortly after her husband, Michael Reynolds, was diagnosed with frontotemporal dementia in 2009. She hopes that others may gain a degree of insight and understanding through this account of her struggles to meet the financial, physical, and emotional challenges that occurred with her bright, talented, and loving husband's passage through FTD.